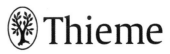

Introductory Guide to Medical Training

From Basic Sciences to Medical Specialties

Manfred George Krukemeyer, MD
Chairman Paracelsus-Hospitals
Osnabrück, Germany

47 illustrations

Thieme

Stuttgart • New York • Delhi • Rio de Janeiro

Library of Congress Cataloging-in-Publication Data

Krukemeyer, Manfred, author.

Introductory guide to medical training : from basic sciences to medical specialties / Manfred Georg Krukemeyer.

p. ; cm.

Includes bibliographical references and index.

ISBN 978-3-13-201211-0 (alk. paper) -- ISBN 978-3-13-201221-9 (eISBN)

I. Title.

[DNLM: 1. Education, Medical. W 18]

R735

610.71--dc23

2015021462

Important note: Medicine is an ever-changing science undergoing continual development. Research and clinical experience are continually expanding our knowledge, in particular our knowledge of proper treatment and drug therapy. Insofar as this book mentions any dosage or application, readers may rest assured that the authors, editors, and publishers have made every effort to ensure that such references are in accordance with **the state of knowledge at the time of production of the book.**

Nevertheless, this does not involve, imply, or express any guarantee or responsibility on the part of the publishers in respect to any dosage instructions and forms of applications stated in the book. **Every user is requested to examine carefully** the manufacturers' leaflets accompanying each drug and to check, if necessary in consultation with a physician or specialist, whether the dosage schedules mentioned therein or the contraindications stated by the manufacturers differ from the statements made in the present book. Such examination is particularly important with drugs that are either rarely used or have been newly released on the market. Every dosage schedule or every form of application used is entirely at the user's own risk and responsibility. The authors and publishers request every user to report to the publishers any discrepancies or inaccuracies noticed. If errors in this work are found after publication, errata will be posted at www.thieme.com on the product description page.

Some of the product names, patents, and registered designs referred to in this book are in fact registered trademarks or proprietary names even though specific reference to this fact is not always made in the text. Therefore, the appearance of a name without designation as proprietary is not to be construed as a representation by the publisher that it is in the public domain.

© 2016 Thieme Medical Publishers, Inc.
Thieme Publishers New York
333 Seventh Avenue, New York, NY 10001 USA
+1 800 782 3488, customerservice@thieme.com

Thieme Publishers Stuttgart
Rüdigerstrasse 14, 70469 Stuttgart, Germany
+49 [0]711 8931 421, customerservice@thieme.de

Thieme Publishers Delhi
A-12, Second Floor, Sector-2, Noida-201301
Uttar Pradesh, India
+91 120 45 566 00, customerservice@thieme.in

Thieme Publishers Rio, Thieme Publicações Ltda. Edifício
Rodolpho de Paoli, 25ª andar
Av. Nilo Peçanha, 50 – Sala 2508
Rio de Janeiro 20020-906, Brasil
+55 21 3172 2297

Cover design: Thieme Publishing Group
Typesetting by Thieme Publishers Group

Printed in India by Replika Press Pvt. Ltd.   5 4 3 2 1

ISBN 978-3-13-201211-0

Also available as an e-book:
eISBN 978-3-13-201221-9

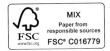

Contents

My Ideal Student

My ideal student, whether male or female, does the following: asks inconvenient questions and learns how to find the answers himself; does his own laundry and cooks his own meals; masters difficult and simple tasks creatively; does not mistake the University for a supermarket; does not solely study for exams; looks forward to semester breaks; is always prepared and knows why; is not a naysayer, and much less a "yes"-man; never settles down if it can be avoided; appreciates a good book once in a while; loves himself, and his neighbor, as himself; does not prohibit anybody from reading certain texts; understands the value and the dangers of the Internet; seeks knowledge, not material gain, and enjoys it; knows that sometimes we have to force ourselves to work, and sometimes go for a walk rather than work; and has trust in his good senses, not in the rankings of journals.

Barbara Mittler, Heidelberg, Germany

Preface

This present book is intended to introduce the reader to the field of medicine. It addresses medical students and persons interested in general information about the medical field, the ways in which the medicine is taught, and the particularities of medical training as a whole.

I became motivated to write this book based on my own studies of health care in the Western world. The many questions and comments I have received from students and publishers throughout the years also helped me conclude that I should impart some of my knowledge in the form of a book meant for the public at large.

Without boundaries, I have tried to write this book so that it reflects how the practice of medicine has become patient-oriented in the Western world. The medical field continues to change, and such changes are necessary to ensure a constant flow of medical diagnostics and therapy—whether they are novel concepts or tried-and-true but forgotten methods. Outdated information is overruled by new insights, meaning that physicians must keep up with such knowledge and, thus, medical education is a lifelong process.

The nomenclature in the fields of pathology and psychiatry has considerably changed in the last 20 years, and a new, unified classification based on international conventions has helped us better understand diseases and improve their respective therapies.

Due to the continuously diverging processes in the medical field, it would be impossible to cover all areas. Social medicine is most certainly an important aspect as are medical informatics and laboratory diagnostics, but I have not covered all these areas. The important topics of tropical medicine and psychoanalysis are only touched upon. Specialty fields also vary country to country; for example, some physicians in the United States specialize in emergency medicine. Public health issues do not have the same significance in Europe as they do in Asia or Africa. The years of education and the way in which would-be physicians are taught—(including the examinations they take)—also differ depending on country, or sometimes even by state—so much so that the extent of variability goes beyond the scope of this book to elaborate on the topic. New areas of study established only in the last few decades, including genetics, immunology, and bioethics, have only been given brief mention. Chapter 1, "Getting Started" and Chapter 3, Section 3.5 "Patient History and Examination" are condensed versions of two chapters taken from my book on the culture of medicine[1].

There are differences between countries in therapies, guidelines, recommendations, pharmacology, and so forth. What is presented here may not be specific to the individual reader's country, so the reader is advised to consult the official standards in their particular region.

Manfred George Krukemeyer, MD

---

1 Krukemeyer MG. Kultur der Medizin. Stuttgart: Schattauer; 2011

Acknowledgments

I would like to thank F. Huebner for all her help in compiling the diagrams in Chapter 2 and the short biographies in the Appendix. I would also like to thank A. Kronenberg for the time she invested in helping me edit and precisely organize the original manuscript. I am very grateful to my secretary, S. Mueller, for typing the manuscript. Many thanks to Ruth Gutberlet, Sherri Damlo, and the team at Thieme Publishers for seeing the manuscript through to production. I would also like to extend my utmost appreciation to V. Krenn, MD, professor of pathology, W. Wagner, MD, professor of radio-oncology, C. Trenkwalder, MD, professor of neurology, B. Christoph, MD, professor of otolaryngology, P. Sukowski, MD, psychiatrist, C. Hendrich, MD, dermatologist, Th. Reisinger, MD, cardiologist, L. Bastian, MD, professor of surgery, T. Zeiser, MD, gynecologist, and P. Barsnick, MD, ophthalmologist, for their accuracy in the painstaking revision of this text.

Section I
What Does It Mean to Study Medicine?

1 Getting Started

Learning is like rowing upstream,
as soon as you stop you drift backwards.

Benjamin Britten

When we ask ourselves what the result will be at the end of the study of medicine, or to what extent the study of medicine has shaped the student, we have to ask these questions in more general terms to find an answer: What does it mean to study medicine, and what must the student learn? Accordingly, this text is divided into two main sections to address these broad questions.

The process of studying medicine begins with learning the science of medicine. The student is introduced to the functions and scientific basics of the body, including chemistry, biochemistry, and physics. In the field of anatomy, which is the study of the topographic allocation of organs and body parts, the student must acquire a basic knowledge about individual tissues and their differentiation; thus, both macroscopic and microscopic anatomy make up part of the curriculum. The student will learn about all of the structures of the body and how they work, including the cerebral cortex, the kidneys, the vascular supply of the eyes, the vascular system of arteries, veins, and the lymphatic system, to name but only a few.

Concurrently, the student will also study physiology, which is a branch of medicine that focuses on the functioning of the body. For example, the student will learn how the inner ear transforms acoustic waves via mechanical vibrations into electric conductivity, how the body controls and centrally monitors the content of the urinary bladder, how the cardiac rhythm works, and will be able to describe the biotransformation of metabolic products in the liver. The student will also study the structure and composition of blood, immune cells (in particular, the function of the immune system), the structure and functioning of the intestines, the sensory organs, inner glands, messenger substances and their receptors, as well as electrolyte, mineral, and water balances. Once the student comprehends how a healthy body functions, where and how organs and tissues are topographically related, the student will learn about diseases, changes that occur in diseased organs on both a macroscopic and microscopic level, as well as the implications for organs and organ systems. Concurrently, the student is also introduced to the numerous medications used to treat disease, focusing on their contents, effects, adverse events, and appropriate dosages.

The focus on anatomy and physiology—which dominates a student's initial introduction to the field of medicine—continues throughout the medical curriculum. This type of two-pillar medicine can be found in the clinical studies in which surgery and internal medicine come together, and they are considered to be two types of the major fields of medicine. Additional subjects of the curriculum include imaging techniques, microbiology, and the examination of patients—in particular, taking an accurate patient medical history: anamnesis.

In another part of the curriculum, the student will study clinical subjects such as internal medicine, surgery, gynecology, pediatrics, neurology, psychiatry, anesthesiology, orthopaedics, forensics, dermatology, and diseases of the sensory organs, among others. By obtaining knowledge in this stepped way, the medical student will learn what the great French philosopher René Descartes has taught us: that we must divide a problem into as many parts as possible to solve the easiest parts, and then work our way slowly to the difficult parts of learning and understanding.

For example, an extraordinary fact the student may learn is that the endothelium, which is the innermost layer in a human blood or lymphatic vessel, contains 10^{13} cells and weighs more than 1 kg. If it is spread out, the vascular endothelium of a human would cover an area the size of 500 m^2; if they are strung together lengthwise, these endothelial cells would reach all the way around the equator! Combine two kidneys and you have more than 4 million glomeruli that total the size of an area of 3.5 m^2. When pulled apart, the length of human deoxyribonucleic acid (DNA) would equal the distance between the Earth and the moon. The student will also learn that gastric carcinoma is a malignant cancer that forms metastases early on, whereas a duodenal tumor occurs only rarely. Other relevant concepts the student must understand include that a fat embolism following an injury may be fatal, that a heparin injection is necessary to avoid fatal thrombosis in older patients who are bedridden but not in children, and that rejection reactions in patients receiving kidney transplantation must be considered while the basic principles of transplantation immunology are of lesser importance in liver transplantation.

Perhaps more importantly, the student will be introduced to preventive medicine, which can be aptly applied to numerous fields of medicine, including oncology. "It would be most important to achieve progress in cancer prevention," stated German physician Harald zur Hausen. "Considering that 90% of all cancer cases have environmental origins, a significant number of those cases should be avoidable" (zur Hausen 1996). Prevention is a practice that medical students will learn. Students who wish to be part of the medical field must recognize that prevention and education are important pillars of public welfare. Despite research that aims to prove its worth and the appeals of international organizations, particularly the World Health Organization, preventive medicine is not implemented worldwide. In many countries, there are those who smoke who are aware that smoking causes the majority of cases of lung cancer. Many Westerners have poor diets, eating foods that contain excessive calories and fat, but it is impossible to offer healthy meals to everyone. Possibly due to "vaccination fatigue" and the "anti-vaxer" movement, infectious diseases are on the rise worldwide. Therefore, it is important to emphasize to medical students the importance of explaining to and educating their patients about the importance of physical education, including regular exercise, the value of dental hygiene, vaccinations, and proper nutrition, particularly because these concepts are sometimes neglected by educators at all institutional levels.

Despite the successes within theoretical and clinical medicine, there are shortcomings that must be remedied and should be emphasized to students wishing to enter the medical profession. For example, biologist and science journalist Ulrike Gebhardt (2010) takes issue with the effectiveness and safety of new medications in children. In Germany, approximately 30% of medications prescribed to children 12 to 16 years of age are not approved for the pediatric population. Off-label use is inversely proportional to patient age: a 60% increase in infant use and 80% increase in newborn use. She explains that it becomes difficult to recommend an appropriate dosage of a drug if that drug has never before been tested on children of that particular age. In clinical studies it is crucial to have a reference group, however, what parent wants their child to be part of a medical trial when the point of the scientific research is to answer a research question, not to consider what care is best for the patient?

Without having learned how the body functions, one will not understand how pathologic changes can develop in the body and the individual organs. One will not understand why a child and an elderly person are not likely to benefit from the same dosage of medication. Anyone who has not learned how to regularly auscultate heart sounds cannot recognize and hear the pathologic changes that can occur in the heart. Without having seen and palpated the fragility of the medial meniscus of the knee joint, as a doctor one would not be able to provide patients with the best possible care. Anyone who cannot locate the ganglia within the central nervous system and is unaware of their interactions will never truly understand the concepts behind therapeutic options for Parkinson's disease. Without having held and felt the spleen in one's hands during macroscopic anatomy, one cannot fully comprehend the fragility of this organ or may not understand why it may cause fatal bleeding in an accident. Anyone who has not learned to examine the hip joint will not recognize the pathologic change in the hip of a child.

The student must also learn how to diagnose and treat internal diseases as part of internal medicine, the conservative part of medical science. In addition to the traditional subjects—those subjects considered to be the backbone of medical education—the medical curriculum typically includes the preclinical concepts of sociology, medical history, and psychology, as well as clinical concepts relating to biomathematics, occupational medicine, pain therapy, dentistry, stomatology, and orthodontics.

A diagnostic eye is mandatory for becoming a physician, and is defined as the ability to recognize diseases in order to adequately respond to them. It also means having the correct judgment and capacity to communicate diagnoses to patients and accompany them on their path through therapy. Many top-class, internationally recognized physicians are unable to share a diagnosis with a patient using layperson's terms. Some professors are also incapable of giving a stimulating lecture, instead monotonously reading from a script because they are unable to speak in front of students, or their patients. These people are incapable of enthralling their students or connecting with their patients. Thus, physicians must apply their diagnostic eye in order to communicate appropriately with the patient, describe diagnoses in a coherent and simple way, and recommend and carry out the best possible care for their patients.

The patient must believe in the physician; faith is an important aspect of therapy. The patient must also have faith in themselves, their subjective reality, and in the physician's medical judgment. Electronic health record systems and other novel, high-tech medicine should not be equated with bad medicine. However, physicians should never forget how to speak to the patient—and, more importantly, to speak with the patient!

The physician–patient relationship means that the physician and the patient establish a fiduciary bond that forms the foundation of effective communication between two people. Language, dialog, sensitivity, compassion, and communication between the physician and patient are vital to the relationship and to the physician's ability to accurately diagnose the patient and recommend potential treatments. The patient meets the physician with confidence if he or she believes that the physician is medically proficient, is able to build trust and rapport with them, and is able to provide optimum support. In this respect, the physicians' demeanor, language, and way of showing that they are willing to help are significant. Mere language skills, which are always mandatory, will still lead to a loss of trust without the investment of time, the building of trust, and the willingness to respond to the patient. The physician must also learn to recognize what the patient needs, which requires that the physician understand the patient. Perhaps the patient is fearful of being alone with their illness. The hospital is an anonymous place—a building made of concrete, neon lights, and sterile colors exuding coldness. The patient lies in their room, by themselves or with people they have never met before. Going to the hospital, not knowing what to expect, what they will have to endure, and knowing that they are at the mercy of clinical apparatus may be distressing to many patients. The student who wishes to enter the medical field must be aware of this.

The medical student must be keenly aware that diseases may be related to life-changing events. A healthy physician–patient relationship is extremely valuable for recognizing these types of life changes. To that end, Thomas H. Holmes and Richard H. Rahe (1967) developed a life-event questionnaire to evaluate when life changes cause diseases. In their research, they found that in 100% of study respondents, the death of a spouse caused stress-related disease. In the case of divorce, separation from a partner, or death of a close relative, more than 60% of study respondents also experienced stress-related disease. Performance breakdown—whether it be a student failing school, a failure in sports, or a failure at work—has the potential to cause pressure and tension, possibly leading to high blood pressure, nervousness, irritability, sleeplessness, or cardiac rhythm disorders, among other ailments. *This* is what is referred to as the subjective state, which needs to be recognized by the physician.

And the physician can influence the patient's subjectivity. For example, a patient will immediately perceive whether the physician is rushed for time. The patient is looking to the physician for honesty, understanding, benevolence, and compassion, among other attributes, and the willingness to focus on them during their office visit.

People experience disease in many different ways. Some may be ashamed; others would prefer not to talk about it; while others may desire empathy. Others still may be open and willing to discuss their condition. Every human experiences a disease in a unique and individual manner. I remember a case from my clinical internship in which two women were both diagnosed with breast cancer and both underwent mastectomy. One woman was thankful that she had come through this difficult surgery and hoped that there were no metastases left; by contrast, the second woman was terribly distraught and did not feel feminine any longer and wanted to put an end to her life. Here was the same disease in two different humans who had two wildly different reactions. But what about the physician? The physician must respect the patient's situation. Sometimes there is even a place for humor. Physicians must meet the patient with sensitivity and always maintain compassion. Empathy for the patient and understanding of the disease are important. Conversely, the physician–patient relationship breaks down if mutual respect and understanding are whittled away due to lack of treatment compliance from the patient.

Physicians must often work as if on an assembly line, whether it is in the operating room or in the outpatient clinic. Electrocardiography (ECG) must be obtained, sonography results evaluated, and endoscopies performed. Somatic complaints must be ruled out. We perform differential diagnoses. We confer with other colleagues. We read the latest medical literature, all to fix the patient. But we have to remember that an ill person is not like a broken machine—he or she is a fellow human being in need of help and care.

The medical student must be aware that it is as important to study and master the science of medicine as it is to understand the difference between the "real world" and that of academia. Many university physicians and researchers may start out with enthusiasm and high expectations, but then their dreams evaporate and hopes go unfulfilled. The university can be treacherous ground on which it is easy to slip and fall. Students who practice beyond the academic setting have opportunities to put their ideas and dreams of improved medicine and adequate patient care into practice, but this will only be possible if students have a positive outlook into the future and a well-founded knowledge of medicine.

By the time of graduation, the medical student should understand the physiology and pathology of the human body, as well as available therapies, and, in turn, be able to discern and apply such knowledge to themselves and the environment. In addition, the medical student must be aware of the great responsibility that comes with being a physician. The Hippocratic Oath, attributed to Hippocrates, an ancient Greek physician living on the island of Kos, expresses the importance of medical agency, power of judgment, and ethics. It is one of the oldest oaths in human history, obliging the physicians to sensibly apply the teachings they have learned to patient care. The prospective physician must also learn to think critically of themselves and the world around them. For example, the Hippocratic Oath states that a physician can only prescribe what has a beneficial effect. How relevant this 2,000-year-old oath is! "Not the possession of knowledge, but power of judgment makes the difference," says the great philosopher Karl Jaspers. "Knowledge alone does not help, but the ability to find the necessary knowledge everywhere through one's own initiative, the ability to use one's own mind to grasp things. This ability is not acquired through studying the subject matter but being exposed to living research" (Jaspers 1961).

2 General Terms

*Happiness is the only thing
that doubles,
when you share it.*

Albert Schweitzer

Universities impart a theoretical and practical education to medical students. When starting their medical training, the student learns about medical science, therapies, the results and consequences of surgical procedures, vaccinations (or lack of), and chronic conditions, among many other topics. Medical studies comprise lectures, seminars, and internships, studying specialized medical literature, scientific work, and the bedside practicing of diagnosis and therapy.

In some circles, medical education is considered part of the natural sciences, although there is a never-ending philosophical discussion as to whether medicine is also a social science. Ultimately, medicine is about obtaining knowledge that can be used to help treat fellow human beings.

In addition to learning facts and applying one's knowledge of such facts, it is essential to stick to precise scientific procedures when studying medicine. It is important to learn the fundamentals and understand the basic principles of scientific procedures—these are basic principles that recur during the student's education and throughout his or her entire medical career.

2.1 Particularities of Medical Training

Studying medicine requires learning by heart. Other subjects may require abstract thinking, such as mathematics, or discussions about the nature of things, such as religious studies and philosophy. Medicine—like other sciences—focuses on *facts*. The anatomic structures of the blood supply of the adrenal gland, the muscles of the upper arm, and the layers of the heart remain unchanged. Hence, medicine requires the memorization of facts. This is true for anatomy, pathology, and every other field of medicine.

Medical knowledge changes over the course of time—the concept of disease is a prime example! In ancient times, disease was interpreted as a twist of fate, a divine or spiritual punishment sent from the gods. For this reason, the first healers—today we might call them shamans—belonged to the priesthood. In general, they used prayers and offerings, as well as dietary and medicinal measures, to "expel" the divine punishment. Hippocrates, an ancient Greek physician who we credit with authoring the famous Hippocratic Oath, was one of the first people to consider diseases as having natural—not supernatural—causes, arguing that disease was related to lifestyle, diet, and other environmental root causes. Later, in the seventeenth century, the concept of disease began to evolve when the English physician Thomas Sydenham—called the "English Hippocrates" by some—discovered that external agents cause disease.

Two centuries later, the French physiologist Claude Bernard suggested that humankind itself creates its diseases. Diseases were not caused by divine and supernatural wrath but instead humans were at the center of disease and its course. This was an expression of the era of Enlightenment in Europe at the time, which was, in general, represented by the German philosopher Immanuel Kant and the French philosopher René Descartes.

Today, we also know that some people become ill because of behavior, habits, and lifestyle. For example, smoking, consuming alcohol, poor dietary choices, and leading a sedentary lifestyle are causes of many diseases. Many times these are choices we consciously make. Through his sociomedical research, the German physiologist Hans Schaefer discovered that most diseases are related to a person's genetics and the impact of that individual's social environment. He rightly points out that we may not be aware of the actual diseases and their causes; patients may not recognize the "silent killers"—those long-standing chronic processes that go unnoticed, such as high blood pressure, and their consequences (Schaefer 1979).

We must maintain balance in life, a balance that is referred to in medical terms as homeostasis. Chinese medicine calls it internal harmony. This harmony also manifests itself in the functional processes of organs (below, I will discuss the individual organs and diseases as part of the medical specialty fields) and, bearing in mind that the human body is made up of more than 70×10^{12} cells, it is important to develop an understanding of harmony within the body—without harmony, functional interactions between the organs are impossible.

For example, obesity causes *dis*harmony. The articular cartilage in the knee joint, the menisci, becomes impacted to the degree of tissue degeneration. The protecting cartilage wears off during the course of time. Ultimately, bone grinds on bone, causing chronic pain, thus prompting the patient to see a physician. Endoprosthesis may be the only therapeutic option at that point. In another example, short-sightedness involves rays that are refracted by the cornea and the lens of the eye. These rays do not meet on the retina, but instead cross inside the vitreous body, resulting in chronic irritation. A patient with short-sightedness must have this condition corrected. If it goes uncorrected, the eyes will become irritated further, become strained, and cause headaches: there is disharmony here. The heart is the classic example of a pressure-suction pump. The atria fill with blood and are compressed while the ventricles concurrently eject blood. Aortic and pulmonary valves accordingly open and close, as do the mitral and tricuspid valves. A pressure-suction pump can only function properly if one pair of valves opens while the other pair is closed. Harmony is the foundation of the way the heart functions.

This principle continues throughout the entire field of medicine. We must learn to be continuously mindful of the harmony that begins to become apparent during the initial stages of medical training. The qualified physician must learn to recognize disharmony within the patient.

In the area of psychosomatics, lack of harmony is demonstrated by a psychological disorder combined with organ manifestation. I remember a 27-year-old woman who reported chronic constipation without any other outward disease symptom. She had had intestinal spasms for up to two hours a day and suspected some rare disease to be the cause of this discomfort. I took a look at this young woman and she seemed normal in appearance for her age. Her weight was as it should be; her complexion was healthy; she looked happy; she was alert and oriented and did not display any disease symptoms whatsoever other than the reported disorder. Due to her age and sex, I asked her whether she was pregnant and if her menstrual cycle was regular. Pregnancy was ruled out and she confirmed that she had a regular menstrual cycle. I also asked her about drug use, even though she did not give the impression of being a drug user, but she denied any use of drugs. She admitted that she did smoke a cigarette every so often on weekends or when out with friends. I then asked if she had been on a diet lately or had changed her dietary habit. She said no. I then decisively asked her: "Has a family member fallen ill or did a friend or family member die lately?" I had not even finished the question before she began to break into tears and left the room. Later she opened up to me and I referred her to a psychiatrist.

The above case is an example of some sort of physical disharmony, articulated by the young patient. The patient may not know why his or her body reacts the way it does. It is crucial to question the condition and carefully approach the situation. We must learn to obtain a holistic picture of the patient in order to see the reason for his or her state. This includes the demeanor of the patient, their complexion, facial expression, and gait, their entire appearance, odor, weight, and condition of their clothing. If the medical student learns to take all of this in and tries to perceive the patient's balance and imbalances, combining these observations with a solid medical education and factual knowledge, then he or she may become a successful physician.

Diagnosis and therapeutic options also change over time. Dosages of medications have changed and some substance groups have virtually disappeared from the pharmaceutical market. In other areas, definitions have changed. The classification of metabolic diseases has been altered to the extent that what I learned during my medical training is far outdated. For example, the classification of diabetes mellitus has been modified several times in the last few years. Research and development force the medical community to accept new concepts and discard the old. Perhaps this is best illustrated by a metaphor Pope Benedict XVI once used in a sermon: a grapevine will become fruitful only when pruned. Every winemaker knows that. We must nurture and prune a good grapevine for it to produce plentifully. The concept works the same in medicine. We cannot shy away from adopting the new and must have the courage to discard the old.

Today, health is considered to be more than the mere absence of disease. According to the World Health Organization (WHO) constitution, "Health is a state of complete physical, mental and social well-being and not merely the absence of disease or infirmity" (WHO 1946). By contrast, disease is not clearly defined. Different cultures define disease differently and provide different interpretations from philosophical, religious, political, and social points of view.

In many cases, medical knowledge has evolved modularly. There are two aspects to this modular concept: knowledge based on previous medical findings and knowledge made available to the medical community from other fields. The discovery of the circulatory system by the English physician William Harvey is an example of developing medical findings from existing knowledge. William Harvey conducted physiologic experiments, and through this systematic approach he was able to demonstrate that the heart pumps blood to the organs from where it returns to the heart. This discovery revolutionized medicine. However, Harvey based his findings on anatomic knowledge provided by Galen, who gained this knowledge centuries ago by dissecting animals. The English physician Christopher Wren and the German physician Johann Daniel Major developed intravenous injections based on Harvey's discovery. Medical development continues and is based on the knowledge of these forerunners.

We can find examples in many other areas. For example, after the hypobaric chamber was developed by German surgeon Ernst Sauerbruch in 1904, it created the possibility to conduct open thoracic surgery. This invention was a breakthrough in thoracic medicine and allowed heart and lung operations to take place at greatly reduced risk. Bacteria are another example. Following the discovery of bacteria by Antonie van Leeuwenhoek in the 1670s, antibiotics were later synthesized and produced in the twentieth century, after penicillin, the first true antibiotic, was discovered by Alexander Fleming in 1928. Percussion, used in medical diagnosing to this day, is an example of the second modular aspect in which knowledge from outside the medical field is used. The Austrian physician, Joseph von Auenbrugger, had learned from his father, who was a wine merchant, that liquids enclosed in a cavity produce different sounds when tapping the container than enclosed air. Joseph von Auenbrugger applied this knowledge to the field of medicine and was able to diagnose changes within the thoracic cavity by tapping the chest.

Another particularity of medical education is the short "half-life" of medical knowledge. Today, the half-life of facts is approximately five to seven years. In other words, five to seven years after students finish their medical training, the knowledge they acquired is likely to be outdated, yet the physician is only at the beginning of his or her career. For this reason, universities should not only impart the theoretical and practical "armamentarium"—the medicines, equipment, and techniques available to a medical practitioner—but also help medical students understand that practicing medicine responsibly means lifelong studies. Universities should teach different ways to continue medical education after students become licensed physicians—for example, by studying professional publications. Medicine is a discipline that is based on knowledge passed on for decades, if not centuries, but is concurrently characterized by a constant flow of new information and new insights that help create new forms of therapy. Mastering medicine requires the memorization of factual knowledge by the student and lifelong continuing education by the responsible physician.

2.2 What It Means to Be a Physician

I am frequently asked what it means to be a physician. My answer has always been the same. Being a physician means treating a person after a skiing accident at a ski lodge so that the person is still alive when the rescue squad arrives the next morning. Every physician should be able to recognize acute hearing loss, treat myocardial infarction and an asthma attack, position and transport a patient properly and handle bleeds. They should be capable of inserting an intravenous injection, suturing a cut, diagnosing melanoma, intubating, administering pain medication, recognizing psychosis or suicidal tendency, examining the retina with a speculum, treating diabetes, detecting epilepsy or epiglottitis, treating bronchial asthma, indicating a need for surgery, delivering a baby, and issuing a death certificate. In addition to these practical skills, the humane aspect is of utmost importance. The physician is not merely a medical expert. He or she must also apply communication skills and ability to empathize while treating a patient. To borrow surgeon Werner Wachsmuth's words, "Being a physician means giving priority to true humanity, altruism, unselfishness and the willingness to make sacrifices" (Wachsmuth 1985). The patient is not a defective machine but a human being whose core requires support. De facto, the physician does not treat the imbalanced metabolism, a specific infection or a neoplasm, but a sick *human being*. Treatment must be integral. The physician should apply his or her full attention to, and make time for, the patient. Internist Franz Penzoldt (1950) explains it this way: "The moment he enters my room, my physician seems to have only one patient and that is me. I know exactly that I am not the only one and that my case is actually rather harmless, but the physician looks at me as if he was here only because of me and in this moment he really is, bringing along all his experience, skill and humanity."

The work of a physician consists of several reciprocally related processes: comprehending the patient's account of their illness and comprehending the course of the disease. This work is accomplished by studying diseases, examining the patient and their condition, such as skin tumors or ocular changes, and using medical judgment with regard to the disease and patient compliance. These three aspects constitute what it means to be a physician. The art of medicine is applying knowledge to each individual patient.

A physician's fields of activity, in addition to private practice, hospitals and university careers, can include the military, police squads, medical examiners' offices, correctional facilities, pharmaceutical companies, and public health departments, among others. As principal investigators, physicians may supervise medical research. They can work as health managers, controllers in hospital management, consultants for health insurance companies, professional medical associations, public authorities, or for institutions related to public aid.

2.3 Learning Styles and Strategies

There are different styles of learning and every student must find out for themselves which one is best suited to their personality. Learning styles are classified by the senses that are most responsive while learning. There are four basic styles: visual learning (learning by watching), auditory learning (learning by listening), learning by reading and writing (engagement with texts), and kinesthetic learning (learning through practical involvement; also called "learning by doing"). Some theories call the kinesthetic style haptic, meaning that it also includes learning through touch. Other theories may include additional styles, such as communicative learning (learning through conversation), olfactory learning (learning by smelling; e.g., for cases of some bacterial infections), and gustatory learning (learning by tasting). An example of gustatory learning from medieval times, but no longer practiced, is a form of uroscopy: urine was tasted to detect diabetes; if the urine had a sweet flavor, the diagnosis of diabetes was confirmed. Diabetes mellitus, which literally means "passing through like honey," owes its name to this procedure.

Visual learning involves looking at sketches, images, videos, and films, among other mediums. Auditory learning involves listening to lectures and taking part in conversations and discussions. Visual and auditory learning are difficult to distinguish at times, and therefore are often lumped together into audiovisual learning. For example, when watching a video, visual and auditory stimuli are transferred. In addition, visual learning and learning by reading and writing blend into each other, because in both cases the focus is on seeing or reading. Learning by doing, the haptic style, plays an important role in medical training, for example, when palpating cartilage or bones. During my own education, I preferred visual learning and learning by reading and writing. After reading about the subject matter, I wrote excerpts and sketched what I saw, which I then memorized.

For some, learning may be easier when the subject matter is broken into different segments. Thus, for some, it is more effective to learn four times a day for half an hour than once for two hours at a time. I believe that attending lectures is as important as learning from distinguished professors and other physicians. Even if it sounds a little antiquated, studying together, quizzing, and explaining the subject in study groups of three to five students is of great value for most pupils. Furthermore, during the course of their education, students should adopt different learning strategies. This includes work techniques such as marking essential passages of texts, compiling sketches and index cards, using additional sources of information, including Internet resources, smartphone and tablet apps, lexica, journals, and databases. Planning and regularly controlling one's learning progress is also crucial. This can be accomplished in study groups with fellow students or alone by maintaining one's concentration and attention, as well as studying and relaxing in the environment where all of this takes place.

Finally, some concluding remarks about electronic learning (e-learning). Since the late 1990s, the options for Internet-based, interactive, and multimedia learning have been constantly growing. Today, in one way or another, every university has established an e-learning concept for medical education. Provisions include learning software, the distribution of study materials through Internet-based learning platforms, systematic disclosure of specialty areas through the provision of link collections, form and database functions, webinars, and virtual learning groups that meet in a chatroom or online discussion forum where they exchange ideas (these may completely replace former study groups) among many other ways and platforms. An increasing number of case reports, simulations, and digital learning games, so-called "serious" games, are also employed as part of continuing medical education. Many types of interactive learning systems offer case reports from various medical fields with the purpose of systematically preparing students for medical courses, exams, and patient examinations. For example, there can be case studies composed of texts, graphics, animations, photos, radiographs, and electrocardiographic (ECG) findings, as well as audio and video files containing case notes, which provide knowledge about the complexity of a physician's day-to-day practice. While working through the example cases, the bio-medical fundamentals are explained and repeated. Interactive tests enable the student to check on his or her current knowledge. CASUS, KLiFO, INMEDEA, and VoTeKK are German examples. There are similar offerings in other countries, for example HumanSim,[1] CliniSpace[2] or Pulse!![3] in the USA (Graafland et al 2012).

Simulations and learning games should be fun, but most of all they should provide knowledge, make acquired knowledge applicable and re-visable, and help students practice the skills that they have learned. These simulations can be implemented as part of the medical training and continuing medical education, as well as in preventive medicine, rehabilitative therapy, and geriatrics. For example, they can serve as a motivational tool for patients to work toward a healthy diet and lifestyle that includes more physical exercise, for the training of mental and motor abilities, and for strengthening concentration and attention.

Some years ago, e-learning was considered the future of education for the twenty-first century. It was assumed that the classic medical training, that is, attending lectures, learning from textbooks, and teaching at the bedside would be replaced by e-learning. Indeed, Internet-based, interactive, and multimedia learning methods offer some advantages in that they provide students and physicians with continuing education programs and access to learning materials independent of time and space. Learning contents and speed can be adapted to individual style. However, what is missing is direct contact with teachers and fellow students. There is debate as to whether chatrooms and discussion forums can replace study groups. Interactivity and simulations in e-learning can present abstract and complex subjects more vividly than books, but some students may find that studying in front of a screen is more exhausting than studying from books. As a result, blended learning, which is the supplementation and expansion of traditional classroom teaching through multimedia e-learning methods, is advocated today.

In summary, learning software, Internet-based learning platforms and link collections, webinars and discussion forums, case reports, simulations, and digital learning games are welcome as a multimedia complement to classic medical training, but, currently, it is not likely that they

---

1 Available at: www.humansim.com. Accessed April 17, 2015.
2 Available at: www.clinispace.com. Accessed April 17, 2015.
3 Available at: www.breakawaygames.com/serious-games/solutions/healthcare. Accessed April 17, 2015.

will be able to replace it. Just as in the past, students must still memorize anatomic terms and biochemical formulas, pharmacologic dosages, techniques, diagnoses, and secondary diagnoses; they must comprehend individual medical relations and be able to recapitulate them on their own. This has not changed despite the manifold options offered by e-learning.

Everyone who wants to study medicine and become a physician should ask themselves if they could truly offer individual and personal care and assume the role of a partner in the treatment of a patient. Anyone willing to be active and assist patients as an empathetic helper is welcome in the medical community. Extensive medical training, continuing medical education, and the willingness to study for the rest of one's life are fundamentals of the medical profession. The desire to help, the capability for empathy, confidence, and determination are fundamental character traits of a physician.

2.4 Medical Training Facilities and Graduates

There are approximately 2,420 medical training facilities worldwide that educate approximately 389,000 physicians every year for our global population of more than 7 billion people (**Table 2.1**).

Globally, medical educational institutions are spread unevenly. Considerably more than one-third (39%) are located in China, India, Western Europe, and the United States. More than 170 medical educational institutions are located in each of these areas, whereas 31 countries (nine of which are located in Sub-Saharan Africa) have none, and 44 countries (17 of which are located in Sub-Saharan Africa) have only one medical educational institution. The number of graduates also differs considerably. The 134 (or 168)[4] located in Sub-Saharan Africa annually train up to approximately 6,000 physicians, whereas the 173 institutions located in North America produce three times as many. In fact, the 188 institutions located in China graduate 175,000 physicians each year. In relation to the respective populations, sufficient institutions and graduates exist in the Middle East, India, Western Europe, as well as North, Central, and South Americas. By contrast, in South-East Asia, Eastern Europe, and Sub-Saharan Africa, the number of institutions and graduates is lacking (**Fig. 2.1**).

---

4 See the note to **Table 2.1**.

Table 2.1 Institutions, graduates, and workforce by region (2008)[5]

Region	Popu-lation (mil-lions)	Estimated number of schools		Estimated graduates per year (thousands)		Workforce (thousands)	
		Medical	Public health	Doctors	Nurses/ Midwives	Doctors	Nurses/ Midwives
Asia							
China	1,371	188	72	175	29	1,861	1,259
India	1,230	300	4	30	36	646	1,372
Other	1,075	241	33	18	55	494	1,300
Central	82	51	2	6	15	235	603
High-income Asia-Pacific	227	168	26	10	56	409	1,543
Europe							
Central	122	64	19	8	28	281	670
Eastern	212	100	15	22	48	840	1,798
Western	435	282	52	42	119	1,350	3,379
Americas							
North America	361	173	65	19	74	793	2,997
Latin America/ Caribbean	602	513	82	35	33	827	1,099
Africa							
North Africa/ Middle East	450	206	46	17	22	540	925
Sub-Saharan Africa[a]	868	134	51	6	26	125	739
World	7,036	2,420	467	389	541	8,401	17,684

Note: [a] The Sub-Saharan African Medical School Study finds 168 medical schools in the region in 2010 (http://www.samss.org/; accessed April 18, 2015).

5 Frenk J, Chen L, Bhutta ZA, et al. Health professionals for a new century: transforming education to strengthen health systems in an interdependent world. Lancet. 2010;376(9756):1923–1958. *The Lancet* by LANCET PUBLISHING GROUP. Reproduced with permission of LANCET PUBLISHING GROUP in the format Book via Copyright Clearance Center.

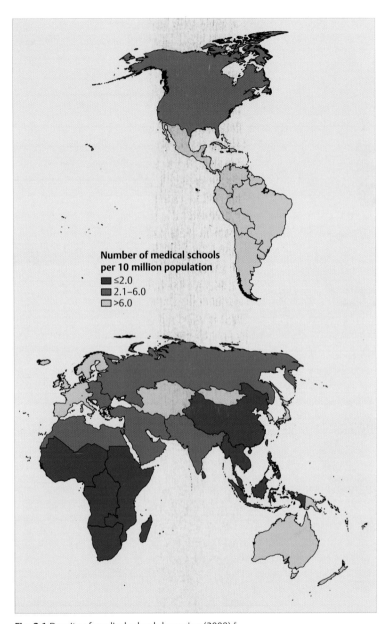

Fig. 2.1 Density of medical schools by region (2008).[6]

6 Frenk J, Chen L, Bhutta ZA, et al. Health professionals for a new century: transforming education to strengthen health systems in an interdependent world. Lancet. 2010;376(9756):1923–1958. *The Lancet* by LANCET PUBLISHING GROUP. Reproduced with permission of LANCET PUBLISHING GROUP in the format Book via Copyright Clearance Center.

Many countries, including some with medium and high incomes, do not educate a sufficient number of physicians to cover their own needs.

During the last 10 years, the increase in the number of medical graduates within the countries of the Organisation for Economic Co-operation and Development (OECD) has varied. The following numbers do not reflect how many graduates were nonresidents who returned to their home countries after graduation. Between 2000 and 2011, Denmark, Portugal, and the Czech Republic had the largest increase of medical graduates per 100,000 inhabitants. There was an increase by 8.45 graduates per 100,000 inhabitants (from 8.37 to 16.82) in Denmark, by 6.28 (from 5.91 to 12.19) in Portugal, and by 6.05 (from 7.86 to 13.91) in the Czech Republic. The OECD average rose from 8.65 graduates per 100,000 inhabitants in 2000 to 10.56 in 2011 (+1.91). However, in some countries, the number of medical graduates decreased. At the top of the list is Slovakia by 2.31 (from 10.80 to 8.49), Spain by 1.53 (from 10.49 to 8.96), and Switzerland by 1.12 (from 10.52 to 9.40) medical graduates per 100,000 inhabitants (**Fig. 2.2**).

Thus, 2,420 medical educational institutions worldwide do not train sufficient numbers of physicians to cover our global needs. Therefore, additional institutions must be created and the number of medical graduates in the existing institutions must increase. Furthermore, the equipment at many institutions must be improved and modernized and, in many places, medical education, as well as continuing medical education for specialty areas, must be adapted to the medical needs of the local population.

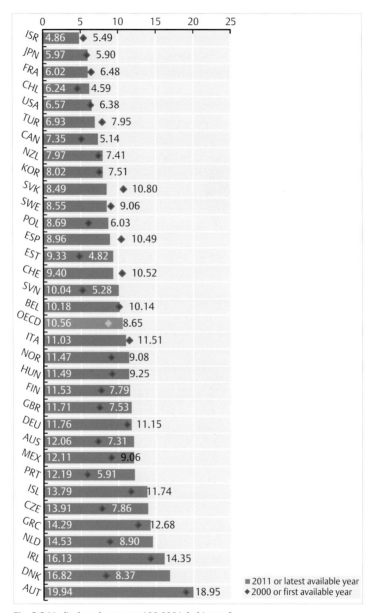

Fig. 2.2 Medical graduates per 100,000 inhabitants.[7]

---

7 Cf. OECD. Doctors. In: OECD Factbook 2014: Economic, Environmental and Social Statistics. Paris: OECD Publishing; 2014:249. Available at: http://www.oecd-ilibrary.org/economics/oecd-factbook_18147364. Accessed November 10, 2014.

2.5 Physicians in Numbers

According to estimates of the WHO, approximately there are 9.6 million physicians worldwide. **Fig. 2.3** displays their global distribution.

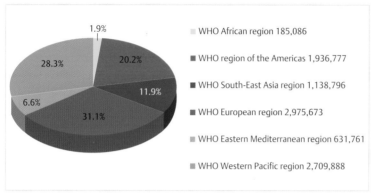

WHO African region 185,086

WHO region of the Americas 1,936,777

WHO South-East Asia region 1,138,796

WHO European region 2,975,673

WHO Eastern Mediterranean region 631,761

WHO Western Pacific region 2,709,888

Fig. 2.3 Estimated number and prevalence of physicians.[8]

This implies a density of physicians as displayed in **Table 2.2**.

Table 2.2 Density of physicians (2006–2013)[9]

WHO region	Density[a]
African region	2.6
Region of the Americas	20.8
South-East Asia region	5.9
European region	33.1
Eastern Mediterranean region	11.4
Western Pacific region	15.3
World	14.1

[a] per 10,000 population.

The largest number of physicians can be found in those areas of the world with the lowest number of cases of illness, whereas smaller numbers of physicians reside in the areas with the largest number of disease

8 Cf. WHO. Global Health Observatory Data Repository: welcome to global health workforce statistics. Available at: http://apps.who.int/gho/data/node.main.HWF?lang=en. Accessed November 10, 2014. The most recent data available for the individual countries was used for the calculation. It is explicitly based on estimation because valid data were available only for a small number of countries and some data are from previous years.
9 Cf. WHO. World Health Statistics 2014. Part III: Global Health Indicators. Geneva: World Health Organization; 2014:138. Available at: http://www.who.int/gho/publications/world_health_statistics/EN_WHS2014_Part3.pdf?ua=1. Accessed November 10, 2014.

cases; thus, many of the inhabitants of these areas do not receive proper (or sometimes any) medical care.

Numbers are available that show those physicians who are in the medical profession for many OECD countries, and partly also for Brazil, China, India, Indonesia, Russia, and South Africa (**Table 2.3**).

Table 2.3 Practicing physicians, professionally active physicians, and physicians licensed to practice medicine (2012[a])[10]

Country	Practicing physicians	Density[b]
Australia	75,258	3.31
Austria	41,268	4.90
Belgium	32,583	2.93
Brazil	355,006	1.84
Canada	86,365	2.48
China	2,138,836	1.55
Czech Republic	38,624	3.67
Denmark	19,232	3.48
Estonia	4,343	3.28
France	201,811	3.08
Germany	318,887	3.96
Hungary	30,641	3.09
Iceland	1,144	3.57
India	883,812	0.71
Indonesia	76,523	0.31
Ireland	12,450	2.71
Israel	25,733	3.25
Italy	229,445	3.85
Japan	292,039	2.29
Korea	104,114	2.08
Luxembourg	1,489	2.80
Mexico	253,486	2.17
New Zealand	11,968	2.70
Norway	21,238	4.23
Poland	85,025	2.21
Russian Federation	703,200	4.91
Slovenia	5,228	2.54
South Africa	38,444	0.73
Spain	178,833	3.82
Sweden	37,063	3.92
Switzerland	31,313	3.92
United Kingdom	175,229	2.75
United States	767,782	2.46

10 Cf. OECD. StatExtracts/Health/Health Care Resources/Physicians. Available at: http://stats.oecd.org/. Accessed November 10, 2014.

Table 2.3 (continued)

Country	Profession-ally active physicians	Density[b]	Country	Physicians licensed to practice	Density[b]
Australia	79,653	3.51	Australia	91,504	4.03
Canada	87,306	2.50	Belgium	55,666	5.00
Denmark	20,547	3.72	Canada	93,347	2.68
Finland	17,790	3.29	Chile	30,321	1.74
France	217,082	3.32	Denmark	29,831	5.40
Germany	348,695	4.34	Estonia	5,882	4.43
Greece	69,435	6.24	Finland	26,367	4.87
Iceland	1,144	3.57	Germany	459,021	5.71
Ireland	14,498	3.16	Hungary	49,613	5.00
Israel	25,078	3.17	Iceland	2,261	7.05
Italy	246,593	4.14	Ireland	18,167	3.96
Japan	300,664	2.36	Israel	32,776	4.14
Luxembourg	1,656	3.12	Italy	380,074	6.38
Netherlands	52,295	3.13	Korea	127,963	2.56
New Zealand	12,017	2.71	Luxembourg	2,117	3.99
Norway	24,453	4.87	Netherlands	65,568	3.93
Poland	92,817	2.41	New Zealand	14,280	3.22
Slovak Republic	18,193	3.36	Norway	27,869	5.55
			Poland	137,109	3.56
Slovenia	5,425	2.64	Portugal	43,123	4.10
Spain	190,833	4.08	Spain	228,917	4.89
Sweden	39,023	4.13	Sweden	57,218	6.01
Switzerland	31,858	3.98	United Kingdom	236,227	3.71
Turkey	129,772	1.73			
United States	809,492	2.60	United States	1,004,635	3.22

Definitions: Practicing physicians provide services directly to patients. Professionally active physicians include practicing physicians and other physicians for whom their medical education is a prerequisite for the execution of the job. Physicians licensed to practice include practicing and other (nonpracticing) physicians who are registered and entitled to practice as health care professionals.
Notes: [a] 2012 or latest available year.
              [b] per 1,000 population.

In the year 2011, on average, more than three practicing physicians for every 1,000 inhabitants were available in OECD countries. The largest number of physicians was found in Greece, with 6.14 practicing physicians per 1,000 inhabitants, followed by Austria with 4.83 practicing physicians per 1,000 inhabitants. Chile, Turkey, Korea, and Poland were the least densely populated areas of practicing physicians among OECD countries; there were calculated to be between 1.58 and 2.19 practicing physicians per 1,000 inhabitants in these countries (**Fig. 2.4**).

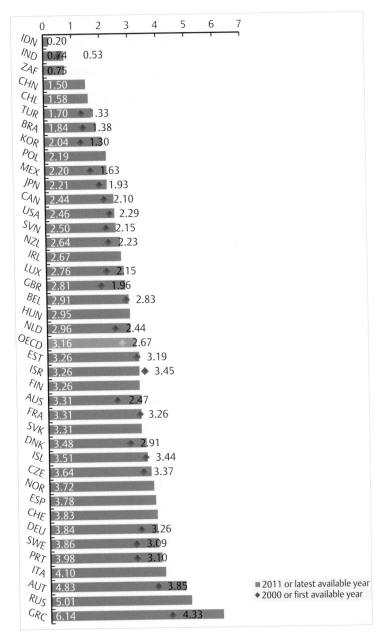

Fig. 2.4 Practicing physicians per 1,000 inhabitants.[11]

11 Cf. OECD. Doctors. In: OECD Factbook 2014: Economic, Environmental and Social Statistics. Paris: OECD Publishing; 2014:249. Available at: http://www.oecd-ilibrary.org/economics/oecd-factbook_18147364. Accessed November 10, 2014.

Between 2000 and 2011, the number of practicing physicians per 1,000 inhabitants rose in all OECD countries, from an average of 2.67 physicians in 2000 to 3.16 in 2011. Israel is the only exception, with the number of practicing physicians decreasing from 3.45 per 1,000 inhabitants in 2000 to 3.26 in 2011. The largest increase in practicing physicians was found in Greece with 1.81, followed by Austria with 0.98, and Portugal with 0.88 additional practicing physicians per 1,000 inhabitants. The number of practicing physicians has also increased in those countries with low initial numbers, such as Turkey, Korea, and Mexico. In France, Estonia, Iceland, and Belgium, the number of physicians per capita has remained nearly unchanged between 2000 and 2011.

In 2012, an average of 56% of physicians practicing in OECD countries were male and 44% were female. In 1990, the proportion of female physicians was only 29%;[12] 10 years later it was already 38%.[13] In Eastern European OECD countries, as well as in Finland, the share of female physicians is markedly above 50%, whereas Japan and Korea are both found at the bottom of the list (with 19.6% and 21.6%, respectively).[14]

In the last decades, the ratio between general practitioners and medical specialists in OECD countries has shifted in favor of medical specialists. The number of medical specialists has increased to the extent that fewer than one-third of physicians practicing in the OECD are general practitioners (**Fig. 2.5**). In 1990, the ratio between medical specialists and general practitioners was 1.5:1. In 2011, it had already changed to 2.1:1.[15] In Central and Eastern European countries, Greece, the United States, Israel, and Korea this ratio is particularly in favor of medical specialists. Only in Ireland are there more general practitioners than medical specialists. In Portugal, Australia, France, and Canada, the ratio is relatively balanced: general practitioners account for approximately one-half of the total number of practicing physicians. The increasing specialization of medicine is one of the reasons for this development. Other reasons include higher salaries for medical specialists (in most OECD countries) and the perception of medical specialists having a better social standing than general practitioners.

12 Cf. OECD. Doctors. In: OECD Factbook 2011–2012: Economic, Environmental and Social Statistics. Paris: OECD Publishing; 2011:278. Available at: http://www.oecd-ilibrary.org/economics/oecd-factbook-2011-2012_factbook-2011-en. Accessed November 10, 2014.
13 Cf. OECD. Health at a Glance 2013: OECD Indicators. Paris: OECD Publishing; 2013:66. Available at: http://www.oecd-ilibrary.org/social-issues-migration-health/health-at-a-glance-2013_health_glance-2013-en. Accessed November 10, 2014.
14 Cf. OECD. StatExtracts/Health/Health Care Resources/Physicians. Available at: http://stats.oecd.org/. Accessed November 10, 2014.
15 Cf. OECD. Doctors. In: OECD Factbook 2011–2012: Economic, Environmental and Social Statistics. Paris: OECD Publishing; 2011:278. Available at: http://www.oecd-ilibrary.org/economics/oecd-factbook-2011-2012_factbook-2011-en. Accessed November 10, 2014.

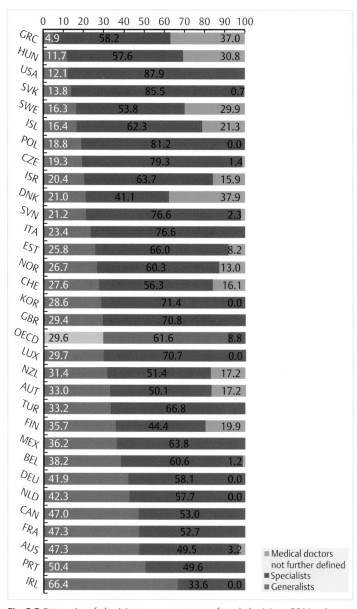

Fig. 2.5 Categories of physicians as a percentage of total physicians, 2011 or latest available year.[16]

---

16 Cf. OECD. Doctors. OECD Factbook 2014: Economic, Environmental and Social Statistics. Paris: OECD Publishing; 2014:249. Available at: http://www.oecd-ilibrary.org/economics/oecd-factbook_18147364. Accessed November 10, 2014.

2.6 Shortage and Migration of Physicians

In 2006, the WHO reported a worldwide shortage of 4.3 million physicians, nurses, and midwives. In 57 countries there are less than 22.8 physicians, nurses, and midwives per 10,000 inhabitants. This number is considered the critical threshold for proper medical care for 80% of all pregnant women, mothers, and children in any given country.[17] This shortage is particularly severe in Sub-Saharan African countries and South-East Asia (**Table 2.4**).

Table 2.4 Estimated critical shortages of doctors, nurses and midwives, by WHO region[18]

WHO region	Number of countries		In countries with shortages		
	Total	With shortages	Total	Estimated shortage	Percentage increase required
Africa	46	36	590,198	817,992	139
Americas	35	5	93,603	37,886	40
South-East Asia	11	6	2,332,054	1,164,001	50
Europe	52	0	NA	NA	NA
Eastern Mediterranean	21	7	312,613	306,031	98
Western Pacific	27	3	27,260	32,560	119
World	192	57	3,355,728	2,358,470	70

NA = not applicable.

In recent years, the number of countries with a critical shortage of medical personnel has grown from 57 to 83. Today, there is a worldwide estimated shortage of 7.2 million physicians, nurses, and midwives; Africa and South-East Asia are still affected by such shortages. In Africa, only Algeria, Botswana, and Tunisia have more than the minimum density threshold of 22.8 physicians, nurses, and midwives per 10,000 inhabitants. In South-East Asia, the number of the affected countries is smaller

---

17 Cf. WHO. The World Health Report 2006: Working Together for Health. Geneva: World Health Organization; 2006:11–13. Available at: http://www.who.int/whr/2006/en. Accessed November 10, 2014.
18 Reproduced, with the permission of the publishers, from WHO. The World Health Report 2006: Working Together for Health. Table 1.3. Geneva: World Health Organization; 2006:13. Available at: http://www.who.int/whr/2006/en/. Accessed November 11, 2014.

but some of these countries are among the most populated, including India with 1.2 billion, Indonesia with 246.9 million, and Bangladesh with 154.7 million inhabitants.[19]

The WHO expects this situation to worsen within the next 20 years, resulting in a global shortage of 12.9 million physicians, nurses, and midwives by 2035, with a considerable lack of physicians, nurses, and midwives in 107 countries.[20]

Physician shortages exist in both developing and emerging countries. Many OECD countries are affected, mainly through their lack of general practitioners and physicians in rural areas. This situation is likely to worsen in future years. The European Commission predicts a shortage of 2 million health care professionals by 2020 in the United States and Europe alone.[21]

The migration of physicians is a considerable factor in the globally uneven distribution of physicians. Physicians move from rural to urban regions and from poor to rich countries, even across continents. One factor that physicians may cite for leaving their home countries is discontentment with living and working conditions. In general, countries that recruit physicians offer financial incentives, better income, continuing medical education, career opportunities, and, frequently, an environment safer than in their home countries.

The phenomenon of the migration of health care professionals is complex and only in recent years has it been systematically explored. Data from some of the OECD countries show that, in some cases, a considerable proportion of physicians or nurses come from foreign countries or were educated in foreign countries (**Table 2.5**).

19 Cf. Global Health Workforce Alliance (GHWA)/World Health Organization (WHO). A Universal Truth: No Health Without a Workforce. Third Global Forum on Human Resources for Health Report. Geneva: World Health Organization; 2014:17–36. Available at: http://www.who.int/workforcealliance/knowledge/resources/hrhreport2013/en/. Accessed November 10, 2014.
20 Cf. ibid., p. 36.
21 Cf. Tjadens F, Weilandt C, Eckert J, et al. Mobility of Health Professionals. Health Systems, Work Conditions, Patterns of Health Workers' Mobility and Implications for Policy Makers. Bonn: WIAD (Scientific Institute of the Medical Association of German Doctors); 2012:1.

Table 2.5 Foreign-trained (or foreign) nurses and doctors in selected OECD countries, based on professional registries[22]

	Year	Number	Share (%)	Sources
Nurses				
Foreign-trained				
Finland	2008	530	0.5	National Supervisory Authority for Welfare and Health (Valvira)
Netherlands	2005	3,479	1.4	BIG Register (Beroepen in de Individuele Gezondheidszorg)
Sweden	2007	2,585	2.6	Swedish National Board of Health and Welfare
United States	2004	100,791	3.5	National Council of State Boards of Nursing (NCSBN)
Denmark	2005	5,109	6.2	National Board of Health, Nursing Adviser
Canada	2007	20,319	7.9	Canadian Institute for Health Information (CIHI) Workforce Trends of Regulated Nurses in Canada
United Kingdom	2001	50,564	8.0	Nursing and Midwifery Council
New Zealand	2008	9,895	22.1	Ministry of Health/Nursing Council of New Zealand
Ireland	2008	37,892	47.1	An Bord Altranais
Foreign				
Belgium	2008	2,271	1.5	Federal Public Service Health, Food Chain Safety and Environment
France	2005	7,058	1.6	La Direction de la Recherche, des Etudes, de l'Evaluation et des Statistiques (DREES), Automatisation Des Listes (ADELI)
Portugal	2008	2,037	3.6	Ordem dos Enfermeiros
Italy	2008	33,364	9.4	Federazione Ipasvi
Doctors				
Foreign-trained				
Poland	2005	734	0.6	Polish Chamber of Physicians and Dentists
Austria	2008	1,556	4.1	Austrian Medical Chamber
France	2005	12,124	5.8	L'Ordre des Médecins
Denmark	2008	1,282	6.1	National Board of Health, Labour Register for Health Personnel

Continued ▶

---

22 Reproduced, with the permission of the publishers, from Siyam A, Dal Poz MR, eds. Migration of Health Workers: The WHO Code of Practice and the Global Economic Crisis. Table 8. Geneva: World Health Organization; 2014:87. Available at: http://www.who.int/hrh/migration/migration_book/en/. Accessed November 11, 2014.

Table 2.5 (Continued)

	Year	Number	Share (%)	Sources
Netherlands	2006	3,907	6.2	BIG Register (Beroepen in de Individuele Gezondheidszorg)
Belgium	2008	289	6.7	Federal Public Service Health, Food Chain Safety and Environment
Finland	2008	2,713	11.7	National Supervisory Authority for Welfare and Health (Valvira)
Canada	2007	14,051	17.9	CIHI—Scott's Medical Database (SMDB)
Sweden	2007	6,034	18.4	Swedish National Board of Health and Welfare
Switzerland	2008	6,659	22.5	FMH Swiss Medical Association
United States	2007	243,457	25.9	American Medical Association
United Kingdom	2008	48,697	31.5	General Medical Council
Ireland	2008	6,300	35.5	Irish Medical Council
New Zealand	2008	4,106	38.9	New Zealand Ministry of Health, Information Directorate
Foreign				
Slovak Republic	2004	139	0.8	Ministry of Health of the Slovak Republic
Japan	2008	2,483	0.9	Statistics Bureau, Ministry of Internal Affairs and Communications
Greece	2001	897	2.5	General Secretariat of the National Statistical Service of Greece
Italy	2008	14,747	3.7	Associazione Medici di Origine Straniera in Italia (AMSI) based on Ente Nazionale di Previdenza ed Assistenza dei Medici e degli Odontoiatri (ENPAM)
Germany	2008	21,784	5.2	Bundesärztekammer
Portugal	2008	4,400	11.1	Immigration Observatory at the High Commission for Immigration and Intercultural Dialogue (ACIDI, I.P.)
Norway	2008	3,172	15.9	Den Norske Legeforening

Globally, the migration of health care professionals is on the rise, particularly the migration from poor to wealthy countries. Consequently, developing and emerging countries burdened most by diseases, and in which health care systems insufficiently provide medical care for their people, lose even more physicians and nurses to highly developed countries. By contrast, due to an ever-increasing population of retirees, health care systems are confronted with an increasing demand for care of patients with chronic and degenerative diseases. For example, the migration of African physicians away from their home countries is highly problematic. According to the WHO, more than 18,500 physicians trained in Sub-Saharan countries (that is, 22.5% of physicians trained in this region) now work in Australia, Canada, Finland, France, Germany, the United Kingdom, Portugal, and the United States.[23] This migration leads to a dramatic decline in medical care for the population in their native countries.

The migration of health care professionals can also be seen within a single continent. **Fig. 2.6** visualizes the migration of physicians across Europe.

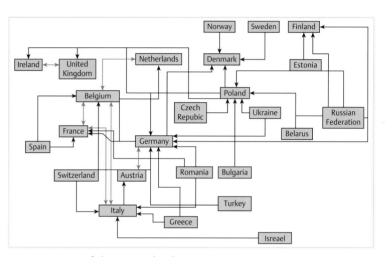

Fig. 2.6 Migration of physicians within the WHO European region (red arrows indicate two-way flows).[24]

Today, in general, Southern and Eastern European physicians and nurses migrate to Western European countries. It is expected that there will also be a shift of health care professionals from Southern to Northern European countries.[25]

When European-trained physicians leave the continent, they usually go to traditional immigration countries, such as the United States, Cana-

23 Cf. WHO. The World Health Report 2006: Working Together for Health. Geneva: World Health Organization; 2006:100. Available at: http://www.who.int/whr/2006/en/. Accessed November 10, 2014.
24 Dussault G, Fronteira I, Cabral J. Migration of Health Personnel in the WHO European Region. Copenhagen: WHO Regional Office for Europe; 2009:16. Available at: http://www.euro.who.int/en/health-topics/Health-systems/health-workforce/publications2/2009/migration-of-health-personnel-in-the-who-european-region-2009. Accessed November 11, 2014.
25 Cf. Tjadens F, Weilandt C, Eckert J et al. Mobility of Health Professionals. Health Systems, Work Conditions, Patterns of Health Workers' Mobility and Implications for Policy Makers. Bonn: WIAD (Scientific Institute of the Medical Association of German Doctors); 2012:161.

da, and New Zealand, where they constitute a considerable portion of the medical profession.[26]

All in all, more health care professionals leave Europe than migrate *to* Europe.[27] The demand for physicians and nurses will grow, but not enough local physicians will be trained or, if trained, they are likely to migrate to other countries. As a result, the competition for well-educated medical staff will be even stronger in the future than it is today. In the worst-case scenario, this migration will cause the number of resident physicians to continue to decline in those countries where health care professionals are already in short supply.

2.7 Five Leading Global Causes of Death

In 2012, 55.8 million people died worldwide, 28.8 million of whom were male and 26 million of whom were female.[28] The five leading causes of death globally in 2012 were the following (**Fig. 2.7**):

1. Ischemic heart disease (estimated 13.2% of all deaths).
2. Stroke (estimated 11.9% of all deaths).
3. Chronic obstructive pulmonary disease (COPD; estimated 5.6% of all deaths).
4. Lower respiratory infection (estimated 5.5% of all deaths).
5. Tracheal, bronchial, and pulmonary cancers (estimated 2.9% of all deaths).

---

26 In 2005/2006, 45,722 physicians trained in Europe worked in the USA, which was 18.3% of all physicians working in the USA. In the same period, 5,267 physicians trained in Europe worked in Canada, which was 38.4% of all physicians working in Canada, and 3,026 physicians trained in Europe worked in New Zealand, which was 45.7% of all physicians working in New Zealand. Cf. Dussault G, Fronteira I, Cabral J. Migration of Health Personnel in the WHO European Region. Copenhagen: WHO Regional Office for Europe; 2009:8. Available at: http://www.euro.who.int/en/health-topics/Health-systems/health-workforce/publications2/2009/migration-of-health-personnel-in-the-who-european-region-2009. Accessed November 11, 2014.
27 Cf. Tjadens F, Weilandt C, Eckert J et al. Mobility of Health Professionals. Health Systems, Work Conditions, Patterns of Health Workers' Mobility and Implications for Policy Makers. Bonn: WIAD (Scientific Institute of the Medical Association of German Doctors); 2012:121.
28 Cf. WHO. Health statistics and information systems: global health estimates 2014 summary tables: deaths by cause, age and sex, by WHO region, 2000–2012. Geneva: World Health Organization; 2014. Available at: http://www.who.int/healthinfo/global_burden_disease/en/. Accessed November 10, 2014.

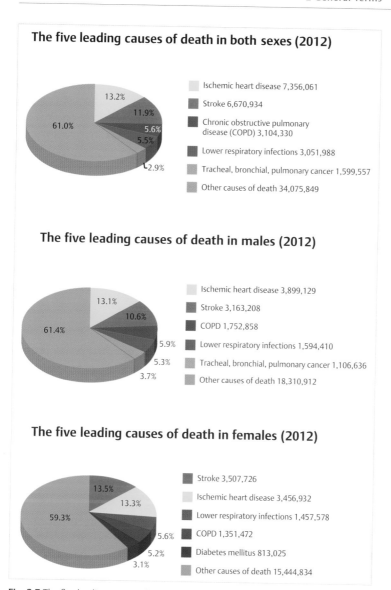

The five leading causes of death in both sexes (2012)

- Ischemic heart disease 7,356,061
- Stroke 6,670,934
- Chronic obstructive pulmonary disease (COPD) 3,104,330
- Lower respiratory infections 3,051,988
- Tracheal, bronchial, pulmonary cancer 1,599,557
- Other causes of death 34,075,849

13.2% 11.9% 5.6% 5.5% 61.0% 2.9%

The five leading causes of death in males (2012)

- Ischemic heart disease 3,899,129
- Stroke 3,163,208
- COPD 1,752,858
- Lower respiratory infections 1,594,410
- Tracheal, bronchial, pulmonary cancer 1,106,636
- Other causes of death 18,310,912

13.1% 10.6% 5.9% 5.3% 61.4% 3.7%

The five leading causes of death in females (2012)

- Stroke 3,507,726
- Ischemic heart disease 3,456,932
- Lower respiratory infections 1,457,578
- COPD 1,351,472
- Diabetes mellitus 813,025
- Other causes of death 15,444,834

13.5% 13.3% 5.6% 5.2% 59.3% 3.1%

Fig. 2.7 The five leading causes of death (2012).[29]

---

29 Cf. ibid.

These five leading causes of death were responsible for 39.1% of all deaths. A total of 14 million people died of ischemic heart disease and stroke, which together caused 25.1% of all deaths, or one out of every four deaths worldwide. Ischemic heart disease and stroke are first and second on the list of causes of death for both sexes. COPD is the third cause of death in males and fourth in females. Lower respiratory infections were the fourth cause of death in males and the third in females. The fifth most frequent cause of death in males was tracheal, bronchial, and pulmonary cancers; it was diabetes mellitus among females.

The five leading causes of death differed only slightly in the WHO regions (**Fig. 2.8**).

In five of the six world regions, ischemic heart disease and stroke are the leading causes of death. In four of the six world regions, lower respiratory infection and COPD are among the leading causes of death. Diarrheal diseases are among the leading causes of death in the WHO regions of Africa, South-East Asia, and the Eastern Mediterranean. Nearly one-half (48.3%) of the total number of deaths in the WHO European region are caused by the aforementioned leading causes of death. In the WHO Western Pacific region, more than one-half of the total number of deaths (52.7%) are also caused by the five leading causes of death. In the WHO European region, two types of cancer are found among the five leading causes of death; tracheal, bronchial, and pulmonary cancers make up the third; colorectal cancer is fifth on the list. In the WHO region of the Americas, Alzheimer's disease and other dementias were the third leading cause of death; diabetes mellitus was fourth. In the WHO Eastern Mediterranean region, preterm birth complications were the fourth leading cause of death on the list. The WHO African region clearly differs from all the other regions: human immunodeficiency virus/acquired immunodeficiency syndrome (HIV/AIDS)-related deaths top the list, followed by lower respiratory diseases, diarrheal diseases, malaria, and stroke.

The global comparison of the five leading causes of death by major cause group gives a differentiated impression (**Fig. 2.9**). In 2012, the leading causes of death included the following major groups:

1. Cardiovascular diseases (estimated 31.4% of all deaths).
2. Cancer/malignant neoplasms (estimated 14.7% of all deaths).
3. Infectious and parasitic diseases (estimated 11.5% of all deaths).
4. Respiratory diseases (estimated 7.2% of all deaths).
5. Unintentional injuries (estimated 6.7% of all deaths).

2.7.1 Cardiovascular Diseases

In 2012, 17.5 million people died of cardiovascular diseases, 8.7 million of whom were male and 8.8 million were female. Totaling 31.4% of all deaths, cardiovascular diseases were the major global cause of death: almost one in every three. People in the WHO Western Pacific region represented nearly one-third (30.7%) of deaths caused by cardiovascular diseases, followed by those living in the WHO European region, where every fourth person died of this type of disease, and by those living in the WHO South-East Asian region, where one in every five (21.1%) deaths was caused by cardiovascular disease (**Fig. 2.10**).

The most frequent causes of death within the major group of cardiovascular diseases were ischemic heart diseases (7.4 million) and stroke (6.7 million). Many cardiovascular diseases can be prevented through a healthy and properly balanced diet, physical exercise, no or moderate alcohol consumption, and not smoking. Cardiovascular diseases are on the rise, particularly in developing countries. The WHO expects the number of deaths caused by cardiovascular diseases to increase to 23.3 million in 2030.[30]

2.7.2 Cancer/Malignant Neoplasm

Cancer/malignant neoplasm is a major group of diseases that represents the second most frequent cause of death. A total of 8.2 million people died of cancer/malignant neoplasms (4.7 million males and 3.5 million females). Of those, 75.6% of these deaths were in the WHO regions of the Western Pacific, Europe, and the Americas (**Fig. 2.11**). Tracheal, bronchial, and pulmonary cancers caused the largest number of deaths (1.6 million) followed by liver cancer (740,000) and stomach cancer (733,500). In males, the leading types of cancer causing death were tracheal, bronchial, and pulmonary (1.1 million), liver (516,700), and stomach (476,000). In females, the leading types of cancer causing death were breast (536,500), tracheal, bronchial, and pulmonary (493,000), and colorectal (333,400).

---

30 Cf. WHO. Cardiovascular diseases (CVDs). Fact sheet no. 317. Geneva: World Health Organization; 2013. Available at: http://www.who.int/mediacentre/factsheets/fs317/en/. Accessed November 10, 2014.

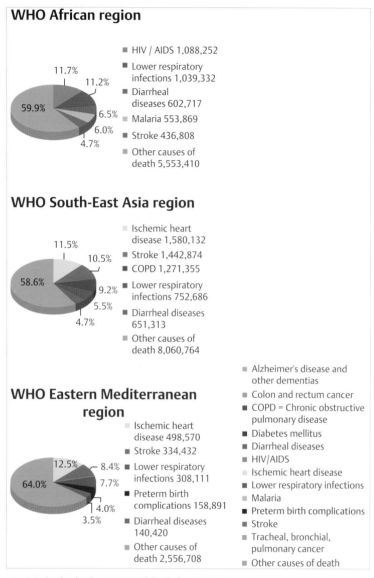

WHO African region

11.7%
11.2%
59.9%
6.5%
6.0%
4.7%

- HIV / AIDS 1,088,252
- Lower respiratory infections 1,039,332
- Diarrheal diseases 602,717
- Malaria 553,869
- Stroke 436,808
- Other causes of death 5,553,410

WHO South-East Asia region

11.5%
10.5%
58.6%
9.2%
5.5%
4.7%

- Ischemic heart disease 1,580,132
- Stroke 1,442,874
- COPD 1,271,355
- Lower respiratory infections 752,686
- Diarrheal diseases 651,313
- Other causes of death 8,060,764

WHO Eastern Mediterranean region

12.5%
8.4%
64.0%
7.7%
4.0%
3.5%

- Ischemic heart disease 498,570
- Stroke 334,432
- Lower respiratory infections 308,111
- Preterm birth complications 158,891
- Diarrheal diseases 140,420
- Other causes of death 2,556,708

- Alzheimer's disease and other dementias
- Colon and rectum cancer
- COPD = Chronic obstructive pulmonary disease
- Diabetes mellitus
- Diarrheal diseases
- HIV/AIDS
- Ischemic heart disease
- Lower respiratory infections
- Malaria
- Preterm birth complications
- Stroke
- Tracheal, bronchial, pulmonary cancer
- Other causes of death

Fig. 2.8 The five leading causes of death, by WHO region.[31]

31 Cf. WHO. Health statistics and information systems: global health estimates 2014 summary tables: deaths by cause, age and sex, by WHO region, 2000–2012. Geneva: World Health Organization; 2014. Available at: http://www.who.int/healthinfo/global_burden_disease/en/. Accessed November 10, 2014.

WHO region of the Americas

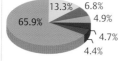

- Ischemic heart disease 854,300
- Stroke 437,875
- Alzheimer's disease and other dementias 318,163
- Diabetes mellitus 304,516
- COPD 280,545
- Other causes of death 4,238,948

WHO European region

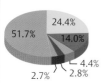

- Ischemic heart disease 2,256,599
- Stroke 1,287,900
- Tracheal, bronchial, pulmonary cancer 405,958
- COPD 259,193
- Colon and rectum cancer 251,830
- Other causes of death 4,769,292

WHO Western Pacific region

- Stroke 2,703,356
- Ischemic heart disease 1,831,039
- COPD 1,097,676
- Tracheal, bronchial, pulmonary cancer 731,680
- Lower respiratory infections 463,315
- Other causes of death 6,133,439

- Alzheimer's disease and other dementias
- Colon and rectum cancer
- COPD = Chronic obstructive pulmonary disease
- Diabetes mellitus
- Diarrheal diseases
- HIV/AIDS
- Ischemic heart disease
- Lower respiratory infections
- Malaria
- Preterm birth complications
- Stroke
- Tracheal, bronchial, pulmonary cancer
- Other causes of death

Fig. 2.8 (continued)

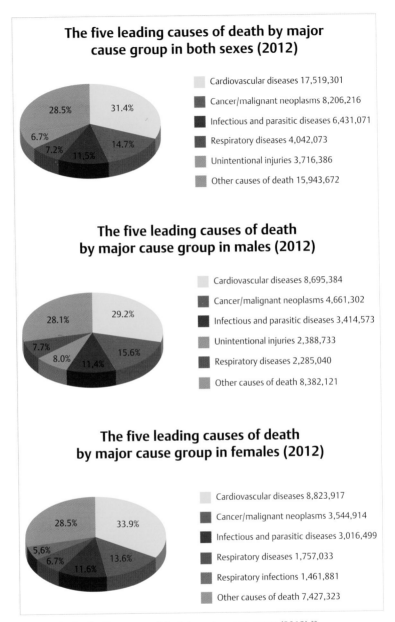

The five leading causes of death by major cause group in both sexes (2012)

28.5%   31.4%
6.7%
7.2%   11.5%   14.7%

Cardiovascular diseases 17,519,301
Cancer/malignant neoplasms 8,206,216
Infectious and parasitic diseases 6,431,071
Respiratory diseases 4,042,073
Unintentional injuries 3,716,386
Other causes of death 15,943,672

The five leading causes of death by major cause group in males (2012)

28.1%   29.2%
7.7%
8.0%   11.4%   15.6%

Cardiovascular diseases 8,695,384
Cancer/malignant neoplasms 4,661,302
Infectious and parasitic diseases 3,414,573
Unintentional injuries 2,388,733
Respiratory diseases 2,285,040
Other causes of death 8,382,121

The five leading causes of death by major cause group in females (2012)

28.5%   33.9%
5.6%
6.7%   11.6%   13.6%

Cardiovascular diseases 8,823,917
Cancer/malignant neoplasms 3,544,914
Infectious and parasitic diseases 3,016,499
Respiratory diseases 1,757,033
Respiratory infections 1,461,881
Other causes of death 7,427,323

Fig. 2.9 The five leading causes of death by major cause group (2012).[32]

32 Cf. WHO. Health statistics and information systems: global health estimates 2014 summary tables: deaths by cause, age and sex, by WHO region, 2000–2012. Geneva: World Health Organization; 2014. Available at: http://www.who.int/healthinfo/global_burden_disease/en/. Accessed November 10, 2014.

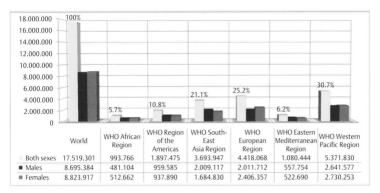

Fig. 2.10 Estimated mortality of cardiovascular diseases (2012).[33]

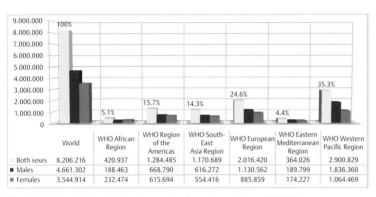

Fig. 2.11 Estimated mortality of cancer/malignant neoplasms (2012).[34]

The global number of deaths caused by cancer is estimated to increase by 64.7% within the next 20 years, from 8.9 million in 2015 to 14.6 million in 2035. All WHO regions are likely to be affected, with little change in the global distribution of cancer-related deaths. Although the absolute number of cancer-related deaths is also likely to continuously increase in the WHO European region, the percentage of those deaths globally is estimated to decrease from 22.8% in 2015 to 18.1% in 2035 (**Fig. 2.12**).

---

33 Cf. ibid.
34 Cf. ibid.

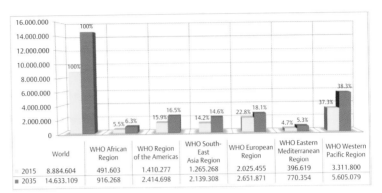

Fig. 2.12 Prediction: mortality of all cancers, excluded non-melanoma skin cancer in 2015 and 2035.[35]

2.7.3 Infectious and Parasitic Diseases

In 2012, three of the five leading causes of death by major cause group were related to infectious and parasitic diseases, comprising 6.4 million deaths, of which globally 3.4 million males and 3 million females died. Almost one-half (49.3%) of all deaths resulting from infectious and parasitic diseases occurred in the WHO African region; the other one-third occurred in the WHO South-East Asia region. This means that nearly four-fifths of worldwide deaths resulting from infectious and parasitic diseases occurred in these two world regions (**Fig. 2.13**).

---

35 Cf. International Agency for Research on Cancer/World Health Organization. International Agency for Research on Cancer/World Health Organization. Globocan 2012: Estimated Cancer Incidence, Mortality and Prevalence Worldwide in 2012/Prediction. © IARC 2014. Available at: http://globocan.iarc.fr/Pages/burden_sel.aspx. Accessed November 10, 2014.

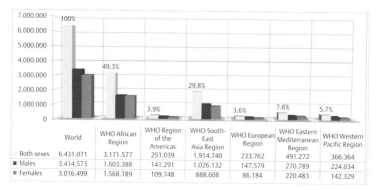

Fig. 2.13 Estimated mortality of infectious and parasitic diseases (2012).[36]

Among infectious and parasitic diseases, HIV/AIDS-related and diarrheal diseases each resulted in 1.5 million deaths; worldwide, tuberculosis alone caused the deaths of 935,000 people.[37] These three infectious diseases are the leading causes of death within this group (**Fig. 2.14**).

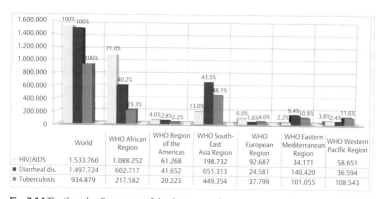

Fig. 2.14 The three leading causes of death among infectious and parasitic diseases (2012).[38]

---

36 Cf. WHO. Health statistics and information systems: global health estimates 2014 summary tables: deaths by cause, age and sex, by WHO region, 2000–2012. Geneva: World Health Organization; 2014. Available at: http://www.who.int/healthinfo/global_burden_disease/en/. Accessed November 10, 2014.

37 Lower respiratory infections were the fourth most frequent cause of death in 2012, with almost 3.1 million deaths (cf. **Fig. 2.7**). They are listed by the WHO in the separate group "respiratory infections."

38 Cf. WHO. Health statistics and information systems: global health estimates 2014 summary tables: deaths by cause, age and sex, by WHO region, 2000–2012. Geneva: World Health Organization; 2014. Available at: http://www.who.int/healthinfo/global_burden_disease/en/. Accessed November 10, 2014.

In 2012, 71% of all HIV/AIDS-related deaths occurred in the WHO African region, where this immunodeficiency disease was the leading cause of death. Globally, HIV/AIDS-related deaths are the sixth most frequent cause of death (1.5 million deaths; 2.8% of all deaths). Since the beginning of this epidemic, 78 million people have been infected with HIV worldwide, and 39 million have died of AIDS-related diseases. In 2005, the number of AIDS-related deaths peaked at 2.4 million. Since then, AIDS-related deaths have decreased by 35%. According to global estimates from the Joint United Nations Programme on HIV/AIDS, 35 million people are currently infected and 2.1 million became newly infected in 2013. The countries of Sub-Saharan Africa are still the most affected: 24.7 million people infected with HIV live in this region, which makes up 70.6% of all worldwide HIV infections. Although the numbers of new infections have dropped in Sub-Saharan African countries by 33% since 2005, the number of people infected in 2013 was still very high at 1.5 million. Areas of Asia and the Pacific are also affected, as 4.8 million people infected with HIV live in these regions. In 2013, a total of 350,000 new infections were estimated to have occurred. The AIDS-related numbers of deaths decreased from 2005 to 2013 by 37%; however, the situation in Indonesia is alarming. The numbers of new infections among people living in Indonesia have increased by 48% since 2005. In other regions of the world, a similar development can be seen. Incidences of new infection increased in the Middle East and Northern Africa by 31% and in Western Europe and North America by 6%.[39]

In 2012, almost 1.5 million people died of diarrheal diseases, 760,000 of whom were below the age of 5 years.[40] Diarrheal diseases are among the leading causes of death in children of this age group. In 2012, diarrheal diseases caused 2.7% of all deaths and were the seventh most frequent cause of death worldwide and the third most frequent cause of death in the WHO African region. In that same year, 83.7% of all deaths caused by diarrheal diseases occurred in the WHO regions of South-East Asia and Africa. It is highly likely that the majority of these deaths could have been prevented through access to clean potable water and better sanitary conditions.

In 2012, 8.6 million people globally had tuberculosis. Of those, 935,000 died (609,000 males and 326,000 females). Globally, tuberculosis is respon-

39 Cf. UNAIDS—Joint United Nations Programme on HIV/AIDS. The Gap Report (and Epidemiology Annex: A36). Geneva: UNAIDS; 2014:8–123. Available at: http://www.unaids.org/sites/default/files/media_asset/UNAIDS_Gap_report_en.pdf. Accessed April 9, 2015.
40 Cf. WHO. Diarrhoeal disease. Fact sheet no. 330. Geneva: World Health Organization; 2013. Available at: http://www.who.int/mediacentre/factsheets/fs330/en. Accessed November 10, 2014.

sible for 1.7% of all deaths and is 13th on the list of the most frequent causes of deaths. If we add to that number the people infected with HIV who also died of tuberculosis, the number of tuberculosis-related deaths increases to 1.3 million for the year 2012. Almost one-half (48.1%) of all tuberculosis-related deaths occurred in the WHO region of South-East Asia, followed by the WHO regions of Africa (23.3%) and the Western Pacific (11.6%). Between 1990 and 2012, the annual number of tuberculosis-related deaths decreased globally by 45%. Alarming, however, is the increasing incidence of multidrug-resistant tuberculosis. In 2012, there were 450,000 global cases of this difficult-to-treat disease and resulted in 170,000 fatalities.[41]

Deaths due to malarial infection represent the fourth leading cause of death in the WHO African region in 2012. Of the global 618,000 malaria-related deaths, nearly 554,000—that is, 89.6%—occurred in the WHO African region.[42] Children younger than 5 years of age in Sub-Saharan African countries were particularly affected.[43]

2.7.4 Respiratory Diseases

In 2012, four of the five leading causes of death by major cause group were respiratory diseases,[44] making up 4 million deaths worldwide (2.3 million males and 1.7 million females). The most frequent cause of death within this group was COPD (3.1 million) followed by asthma (386,000). Nearly three-quarters (71.2%) of all deaths related to respiratory diseases occurred in the WHO regions of South-East Asia and the Western Pacific region (**Fig. 2.15**).

According to WHO worldwide estimates, 64 million people have COPD.[45] In 2012, a total of 3.1 million people died of this pulmonary dis-

---

41 Cf. WHO. Global Tuberculosis Report 2013. Geneva: World Health Organization; 2013:6. Available at: http://www.who.int/tb/publications/global_report/en. Accessed November 10, 2014.
42 Cf. WHO. Health statistics and information systems: global health estimates 2014 summary tables: deaths by cause, age and sex, by WHO region, 2000–2012. Geneva: World Health Organization; 2014. Available at: http://www.who.int/healthinfo/global_burden_disease/en/. Accessed November 10, 2014.
43 Cf. WHO. World Malaria Report: 2013. Geneva: World Health Organization; 2013:63. Available at: http://www.who.int/malaria/publications/world_malaria_report_2013/report/en/. Accessed November 10, 2014.
44 Non-contagious respiratory diseases are distinguished from contagious respiratory infections; they are distinct disease groups.
45 Cf. WHO. Chronic respiratory diseases: chronic obstructive pulmonary disease (COPD). Geneva: World Health Organization 2014. Available at: http://www.who.int/respiratory/copd/en/. Accessed November 10, 2014.

ease, making up 5.6% of all global deaths. Almost 90% of these deaths occurred in countries with low or medium incomes. Causes for COPD include smoking, indoor air pollution (caused from the use of solid fuel for cooking and heating), outdoor air pollution, occupational dust and chemicals, and frequent lower respiratory infections during childhood. The WHO expects COPD-related deaths to increase by 30% in the next 10 years, primarily due to increased tobacco use in many countries with lower and medium incomes.[46]

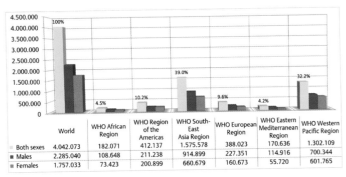

	World	WHO African Region	WHO Region of the Americas	WHO South-East Asia Region	WHO European Region	WHO Eastern Mediterranean Region	WHO Western Pacific Region
Both sexes	4.042.073	182.071	412.137	1.575.578	388.023	170.636	1.302.109
Males	2.285.040	108.648	211.238	914.899	227.351	114.916	700.344
Females	1.757.033	73.423	200.899	660.679	160.673	55.720	601.765

Fig. 2.15 Estimated mortality of respiratory diseases (2012).[47]

Each year 6 million people die as a result of smoking. By 2030, this number could increase to 8 million if tobacco use continues to increase in many regions of the world.[48] Smoking increases the risk of cardiovascular diseases, cancer/malignant neoplasms, and pulmonary diseases such as COPD and asthma. According to estimates from the WHO, 100 million people have died in the twentieth century as a result of smoking. The WHO warns of the possibility that 1 billion people may die of the results of smoking in the twenty-first century.[49]

---

46 Cf. WHO. Chronic obstructive pulmonary disease (COPD). Fact sheet no. 315. Geneva: World Health Organization; 2013. Available at: http://www.who.int/mediacentre/factsheets/fs315/en/. Accessed November 10, 2014.

47 Cf. WHO. Health statistics and information systems: global health estimates 2014 summary tables: deaths by cause, age and sex, by WHO region, 2000–2012. Geneva: World Health Organization; 2014. Available at: http://www.who.int/healthinfo/global_burden_disease/en/. Accessed November 10, 2014.

48 Cf. Mathers CD, Loncar D. Projections of global mortality and burden of disease from 2002 to 2030. PLoS Med. 2006;3(11):e422. (Data taken from: WHO. Global Report: Mortality Attributable to Tobacco. Geneva: World Health Organization; 2012:4. Available at: http://www.who.int/tobacco/publications/surveillance/rep_mortality_attributable/en/. Accessed November 10, 2014.)

49 Cf. WHO. Tobacco. Fact sheet No. 339. Geneva: World Health Organization; 2014. Available at: http://www.who.int/mediacentre/factsheets/fs339/en/. Accessed November 10, 2014.

Other addictive disorders—specifically alcoholism and drug abuse—are also responsible for numerous deaths. In 2012, a total of 3.3 million people died due to alcohol-related causes, making up 5.9% of all deaths worldwide (7.6% of all deaths in males and 4% of all deaths in females were related to alcohol use). Excessive alcohol consumption can cause health issues and may lead to alcoholism, which in turn puts people at increased risks of liver cirrhosis, cardiovascular disease, and some forms of cancer/malignant neoplasms. Between 2005 and 2010, the global consumption of alcohol only slightly increased. It may be true that alcohol consumption is related to the economic prosperity of a country. It is estimated that by 2025 alcohol consumption will increase in the WHO regions of the Western Pacific, the Americas, and South-East Asia. The WHO European region will remain the global leader of per capita alcohol consumption.[50]

According to United Nations Office on Drugs and Crime worldwide estimates, 243 million people in 2012 between the ages of 15 and 64 years—which represents 5.2% of the global population—used illicit drugs, including cannabis, opioids, cocaine, or amphetamines at least once. A total of 27 million people are estimated to be drug abusers, 12.7 million of whom use intravenous forms of drugs. That equates to 0.27% of the global population between the ages of 15 and 64 years. In 2012, an estimated 183,000 people died as a result of drug use. The highest fatality rate—142.1 drug-related deaths per 1 million deaths in the age group between 15 and 64 years—belongs to North America followed by Oceania (77.5). The most frequent cause of death in this population is drug overdose, mainly in cases of heroin use and prescription opioids.[51] Using illicit drugs carries many health risks and can result in a number of secondary diseases. It may result in physical and psychological dependency and the use of contaminated syringes may result in HIV and hepatitis B and C virus infections.

50 Cf. WHO. Global Status Report on Alcohol and Health 2014. Geneva: World Health Organization; 2014:40–48. Available at: http://www.who.int/substance_abuse/publications/global_alcohol_report/en/. Accessed November 10, 2014.
51 Cf. United Nations Office on Drugs and Crime. World Drug Report 2014 (United Nations Publication, Sales No. E.14.XI.7), © United Nations, June 2014. Vienna: UNODC; 2014:1–6. Available at: http://www.unodc.org/wdr2014/. Accessed November 10, 2014.

2.7.5 Unintentional Injuries

In 2012, the fifth leading worldwide cause of death by major cause group was unintentional injury, representing 3.7 million deaths (2.4 million males and 1.3 million females). Almost one-third (31.1%) of all deaths due to unintentional injuries occurred in the WHO regions of South-East Asia, followed by the Western Pacific (21.3%) and Africa (18.7%) (**Fig. 2.16**).

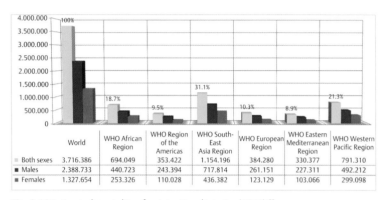

	World	WHO African Region	WHO Region of the Americas	WHO South-East Asia Region	WHO European Region	WHO Eastern Mediterranean Region	WHO Western Pacific Region
Both sexes	3.716.386	694.049	353.422	1.154.196	384.280	330.377	791.310
Males	2.388.733	440.723	243.394	717.814	261.151	227.311	492.212
Females	1.327.654	253.326	110.028	436.382	123.129	103.066	299.098

Fig. 2.16 Estimated mortality of unintentional injuries (2012).[52]

In 2012, 1.3 million people worldwide died in motor vehicle collisions, 693,000 died of falls, and 372,000 people drowned. Another 804,000 people died of self-inflicted injuries and suicides (considered intentional injuries). There is an apparent difference in sex among those who die due to drowning and those who die in motor vehicle collisions: nearly three-quarters of all fatalities related to motor vehicle collisions were male and twice the number of males than females drowned (**Fig. 2.17**).

---

52 Cf. WHO. Health statistics and information systems: global health estimates 2014 summary tables: deaths by cause, age and sex, by WHO region, 2000–2012. Geneva: World Health Organization; 2014. Available at: http://www.who.int/healthinfo/global_burden_disease/en/. Accessed November 10, 2014.

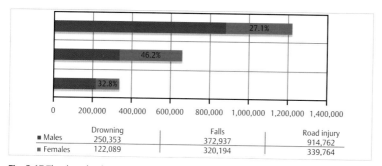

	Drowning	Falls	Road injury
■ Males	250,353	372,937	914,762
■ Females	122,089	320,194	339,764

Fig. 2.17 The three leading causes of death among unintentional injuries, by sex (2012).[53]

The considerably higher number of deaths among males is most likely due to the generally increased willingness to take risks among males, a behavior noticeable in traffic as well as in swimming and (occupational) boating.[54]

2.7.6 Summary

In five of the six regions of the WHO, people do not generally die as a result of contagious disease; most deaths in these regions are due to cardiovascular disease, cancer/malignant neoplasms, and chronic respiratory disease. In the WHO African region, most people die of contagious infectious and parasitic diseases and respiratory infections. In the WHO regions of Africa and the Eastern Mediterranean, 9.8% and 9.1%, respectively, of all deaths are caused by neonatal conditions. In the WHO region of the Americas, neurologic conditions (e.g., Alzheimer's disease, dementia, Parkinson's disease), exceeded only by cardiovascular diseases and cancer/malignant neoplasms, are responsible for the largest number of deaths. In the WHO European region, digestive diseases (e.g., liver cirrhosis, peptic ulcer disease), exceeded only by cardiovascular diseases and cancer/malignant neoplasms, cause the largest number of deaths (**Fig. 2.18**).

---

53 Cf. WHO. Health statistics and information systems: global health estimates 2014 summary tables: deaths by cause, age and sex, by WHO region, 2000–2012. Geneva: World Health Organization; 2014. Available at: http://www.who.int/healthinfo/global_burden_disease/en/. Accessed November 10, 2014.
54 Cf. WHO. Drowning. Fact sheet no. 347. Geneva: World Health Organization; 2014. Available at: http://www.who.int/mediacentre/factsheets/fs347/en/. Accessed November 10, 2014.

WHO African region

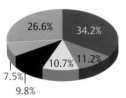

- Infectious and parasitic diseases 3,171,577
- Respiratory infections 1,041,897
- Cardiovascular diseases 993,766
- Neonatal conditions 909,574
- Unintentional injuries 694,049
- Other causes of death 2,463,525

WHO South-East Asia region

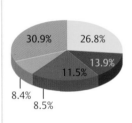

- Cardiovascular diseases 3,693,947
- Infectious and parasitic diseases 1,914,740
- Respiratory diseases 1,575,578
- Cancer/malignant neoplasms 1,170,689
- Unintentional injuries 1,154,196
- Other causes of death 4,249,974

WHO Eastern Mediterranean region

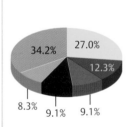

- Cardiovascular diseases 1,080,444
- Infectious and parasitic diseases 491,272
- Cancer/malignant neoplasms 364,026
- Neonatal conditions 362,388
- Unintentional injuries 330,377
- Other causes of death 1,368,625

- Cancer/malignant neoplasms
- Cardiovascular diseases
- Digestive diseases
- Infectious and parasitic diseases
- Neonatal conditions
- Neurological conditions
- Respiratory diseases
- Respiratory infections
- Unintentional injuries
- Other causes of death

Continued ▶

Fig. 2.18 The five leading causes of death, by major cause group and WHO region (2012).[55]

55 Cf. WHO. Health statistics and information systems: global health estimates 2014 summary tables: deaths by cause, age and sex, by WHO region, 2000–2012. Geneva: World Health Organization; 2014. Available at: http://www.who.int/healthinfo/global_burden_disease/en/. Accessed November 10, 2014.

WHO region of the Americas

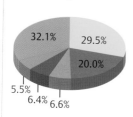

- Cardiovascular diseases 1,897,475
- Cancer/malignant neoplasms 1,284,485
- Neurological conditions 422,550
- Respiratory diseases 412,137
- Unintentional injuries 353,422
- Other causes of death 2,064,278

WHO European region

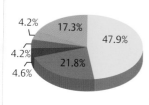

- Cardiovascular diseases 4,418,068
- Cancer/malignant neoplasms 2,016,420
- Digestive diseases 424,445
- Respiratory diseases 388,023
- Unintentional injuries 384,280
- Other causes of death 1,599,536

WHO Western Pacific region

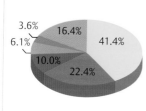

- Cardiovascular diseases 5,371,830
- Cancer/malignant neoplasms 2,900,829
- Respiratory diseases 1,302,109
- Unintentional injuries 791,310
- Respiratory infections 465,237
- Other causes of death 2,129,190

- Cancer/malignant neoplasms
- Cardiovascular diseases
- Digestive diseases
- Infectious and parasitic diseases
- Neonatal conditions
- Neurological conditions
- Respiratory diseases
- Respiratory infections
- Unintentional injuries
- Other causes of death

Fig. 2.18 (Continued)

Section II
What Must the Student Learn?

3 Description of Medical Specialties

I was not a good doctor,
my studies had been too rapid,
my hospital training short,
but there is not the slightest doubt
that I was a successful doctor.
What is the secret of the success?
To inspire confidence.

Axel Munthe

3.1 Anatomy

The word *anatomy* is derived from the Greek *anatome* from *anatemnein*, which means "to cut up." Anatomy itself is divided into several areas. Macroscopic anatomy addresses the body structure and the location of the organs in relation to one another. Microscopic anatomy addresses histology, the science of tissues, and cytology, which is the science of cells. Microscopic anatomy examines human tissue under the microscope and illustrates the individual structures of the various organs.

Cadavers are examined in the anatomy dissection hall or lab. The skin, the individual layers of muscles in the extremities, the vessels in the abdominal cavity, the nerves, and the organs are prepared. Their location relative to each other is evaluated and the anatomic structures are revealed. Based on systematic structures—for example, the tissue layers of the gastrointestinal tract—the student learns about the structure of the organs and other important structures crucial to further diagnosis, particularly when determining tumor stages.

In Ancient Rome, Galen of Pergamon focused on the findings of Greek medicine. At that time, the prevailing theory of medicine was that the four "humors" or bodily fluids (blood, phlegm, yellow bile, and black bile) directly influenced a person's temperament and health. It was not until Andreas Vesalius in the sixteenth century that this ancient idea of medicine was challenged. Galen had acquired his knowledge mainly through the dissection of monkeys and dogs, whereas the approach of Flemish physician and anatomist Andreas Vesalius was different. He is credited with developing the study of human anatomy. In 1543, he published De

Humani Corporis Fabrica (The Fabric of the Human Body), which revolutionized medicine. Other researchers, such as William Harvey and his studies on blood circulation, also shaped the field of human anatomy. In 1628, Harvey published his own revolutionary manuscript, titled *Exercitatio Anatomica de Motu Cordis et Sanguinis in Animalibus* (Anatomic Studies on the Motions of the Heart and the Blood in Living Beings). Through numerous experiments he discovered how the workings of the circulation of blood contradicted the prevailing doctrine. This shows that old traditions were being challenged and new theories were being verified through experiments. It was often very difficult to challenge the old theories, and scientists of the day had to fight hard against them until the evidence just became too strong to refute. From this we learn two things. First, the history of medicine is filled with people's names. Behind diseases, descriptions, and enzymatic processes, we find physicians, clinicians, and scientists who often worked in their respective research fields for decades and perpetuated their names as part of medicine. Second, medicine is subject to constant change. What used to be considered correct and valid scientific consensus may be seen as false and inadmissible today. That which is acceptable today may have been frowned upon decades ago and could have led to an occupational ban. Until a few years ago, stem cell research was mostly ignored, yet groundbreaking developments are now taking place in this field.

It is important that young medical students become accustomed to how quickly these types of changes occur within the medical field. One of the educational objectives of the medical school is for the student to question one's own practice, knowledge, and abilities in order to provide the best care for patients. This education starts with anatomy.

Medicine continues to evolve, so it is crucial to know the anatomy of the human body. Descriptive anatomy serves this purpose by depicting individual organs and structures. It shows us the skeletal system (called the passive locomotor system), including the bones and joints, the muscular system (called the active locomotor system), the digestive system, the respiratory system, the urinary and reproductive systems, the vascular system, the nervous system, the sensory organs, and the layers of the skin. After having systematically studied this part of anatomy, next follows another interesting subject—topographic anatomy. Here, students learn about the exact relation of the individual organs to their environment and neighboring organs. This knowledge can be vital when we want to inject into a vein, not the adjacent nerve. Thus, the vascular supply of the stomach must be well known before surgically intervening, otherwise vascular injuries can easily lead to fatal bleeding. Topographic anatomy alone can impart the function of the basal ganglia, as well as the danger of abdominal injuries or the differing venous drainages of the right and left adrenal glands.

In addition to macroscopic and microscopic anatomy, embryology is an important aspect of anatomy, involving the germination of the ovum and sperm cell and the ensuing development of a new organism. We study the different stages of organ development and learn about the significance of the entire maturation stage, including the danger posed to embryonic development due to radiation, drug use, alcohol consumption, or smoking during pregnancy. The study of anatomy begins with the building blocks of the body. First come cells and the cell body, followed by the nucleus of the cell and its various other elements. We learn about cell division, mitosis and meiosis, and then move on to the differentiated tissues. Surfaces are covered with epithelial tissue, and connective tissue fills the space between tissues and organs. In addition to adipose tissue, we learn about cartilaginous and osseous tissues. We continue with learning about muscular tissue, the functions of muscles, and the voluntary control of muscles via nerves that transmit cerebral impulses. We are introduced to the various muscles and learn that they are categorized as, for example, flexors or extensors and adductors or abductors. The function of the various vessels, that is, arteries, veins, and lymphatic vessels, is explained, as well as the autonomic nervous system, that is, the sympathetic and parasympathetic systems. (We will take another close look at the autonomic nervous system in the physiology section of this chapter.) The skin and its appendages conclude the general anatomy unit.

Anatomy can be taught in varying ways. Generally, in most countries, the curriculum begins with general anatomy, as described above, and is followed by the study of the bones. The student's knowledge about every one of the more than 200 bones in the human body will be tested. Their knowledge about tendons, ligaments, and muscles will also be examined. The class that generally follows will be actual dissection in the dissection lab, a class that takes several months. Its subjects are the extremities, arms, and legs. A second part to the dissection class takes several months and is concerned with the abdomen and abdominal wall, particularly the organs of the upper abdominal cavity (that is, stomach, duodenum, liver, gallbladder, pancreas, spleen), including their topography, the vascular supply of the upper abdominal cavity and the retroperitoneal space, which consists of the kidneys, adrenal glands, ureter and their vascular supply. This part of the dissection class continues with the structure of the back, the vertebral canal, and its pathways, followed by the pelvic organs (in particular, the male and female urinary and reproductive systems), the rectum, urinary bladder, ureter, and male and female pelvic vessels and nerves. Students will learn about the topographically applied anatomy of the neck and about nerves, vessels, and the muscles of the neck and head. They are introduced to the structures of the vascular supply of the eyes, the structures of the ear, the inner ear, and the brain, and the contents of the chest cavity, including the pleural cavities, lungs, mediastinum, and heart. In addition to courses in anatomic dissection, microscopy courses, courses concerned with histology, and embryology courses are offered. Typically, anatomy is taught in 1 to 1.5 years. By then, students should have gained knowledge of the structure of the human body, including its topography, in order to move on to the next step of their medical studies and begin physiology, a field that addresses how the human body functions.

3.2 Physiology and Biochemistry

Physiology is the science of the functions and life processes of the human body. The life processes of the body are based on biochemical functions and sequences. The elemental composition of the body mainly consists of oxygen, carbon, hydrogen, nitrogen, calcium, phosphorus, and a few other elements. The foundation of life is the cell (first introduced in the studies of anatomy and histology). We will encounter Rudolf Virchow and his tenet "*omnis cellula e cellula*" (every cell originates from a cell) (Virchow 1862), which, according to this assertion, determines that physiology is focused on the cells and the interaction of the cellular functions.

Typically, most textbooks begin the physiology units with the functions of the nerve cells (**Fig. 3.1**). It is important for students to understand the cell membrane and the action potential, that is, potassium is found *inside* the cell at a level of high concentration and sodium is found *outside* the cell at a level of high concentration. Sodium entering or potassium exiting triggers the action potential of the cell membrane.

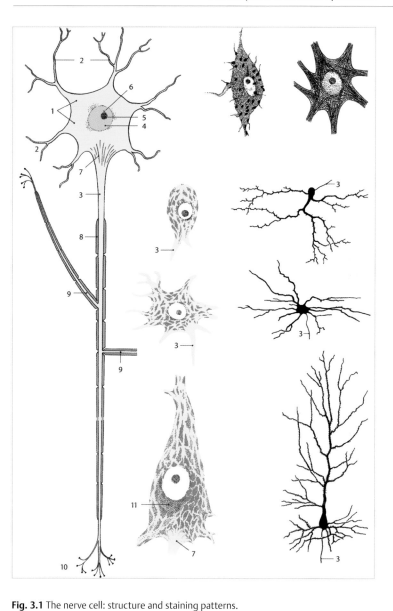

Fig. 3.1 The nerve cell: structure and staining patterns.
1 Perikaryon, 2 Dendrites, 3 Axon or neurite, 4 Cell nucleus, 5 Nucleolus, 6 Barr body, 7 Axon hillock, 8 Myelin sheath, 9 Axon collaterals, 10 Terminal area (axon terminals, or boutons), 11 Melanin, lipofuscin.

This basic function is first explained using the example of the nerve cells, and the concept is then transferred to the functioning of the muscles and the interaction between nerves and muscles. We learn that the action potential in the nerve cell can trigger a muscle to contract. Based on this process, we can explain muscle function, which includes adenosine and myosin bonds and the synergy of the myosin head and adenosine triphosphate (ATP). Thus, we learn about the physiology of nerve cells, neural networks, and the motor systems, particularly the motor end plate.

The science of the sensory organs is part of a subfield of physiology called sensory physiology. It teaches how light is refracted through the cornea into the lens and then transmitted to the most sensitive tissue of the body, the retina. The ray of light is sent from the retina to the central nervous system, which is where the signal is processed and sent on to the visual cortex. We learn about how eye movement and the sense of position are connected. In addition to the organs of hearing and equilibrium, the other senses students will learn about include taste, smell, thirst, and hunger, as well as their interactions.

The heart carries out one of the most vital functions in the human body. The physiology of the heart muscle, the contraction, the Windkessel effect of the aorta, the sensitivity of the coronary vessels, the atria, the pulmonary and aortic valves, the ventricular contractions, and the filling of the atria make up the foundational knowledge required to understand how the human heart functions (**Fig. 3.2**). An electrocardiographic (ECG) study supplies a read-out of the contractions, providing important information regarding atrial contraction, atrial–ventricular conduction time, ventricular contraction, frequency, and rhythm of the heart.

Furthermore, the medical student learns about the function of the vascular system, the varieties of blood supply to the individual organs, the singular supply of the brain or heart via a terminal vessel, the fragility of the venous system (particularly with regard to injuries inside the abdominal cavity), the importance of fluid transport within the lymphatic tissues, and the potential transmission of tumor cells through the lymphatic system.

This unit of study is followed by teachings on respiration and the absorption of oxygen, the barriers between the alveoli and the vascular wall, the capacity of the lungs to expand (and the risks of the same), the release of oxygen throughout the peripheral tissues, and the reliance of the entire body on oxygen, because cell death due to lack of oxygen is irreversible.

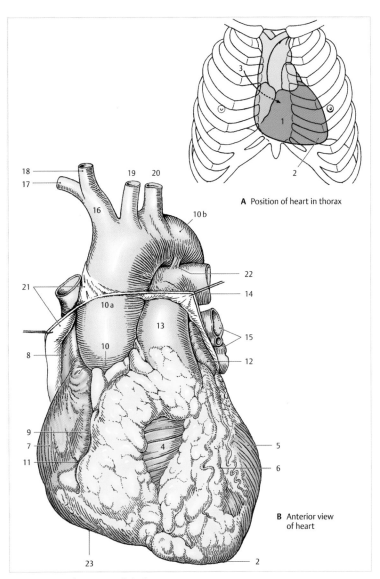

Fig. 3.2 External anatomy of the heart.

1 Heart, 2 Apex of the heart, 3 Base of the heart, 4 Right ventricle, 5 Left ventricle, 6 Anterior interventricular sulcus, 7 Right atrium, 8 Superior vena cava, 9 Right auricle, 10 Root of the aorta, 10a Ascending aorta, 11 Coronary sulcus, 12 Left auricle, 13 Pulmonary trunk, 14 Pulmonary artery, 15 Left pulmonary veins, 16 Brachiocephalic trunk, 17 Right subclavian artery, 18 Right common carotid artery, 19 Left common carotid artery, 20 Left subclavian artery, 21 Pericardium, 22 Ligamentum arteriosum, 23 Right border

The transport medium inside the vessels is blood. The student learns about the blood cells: the red blood cells (erythrocytes) without, and the white blood cells (leukocytes) with a nucleus.

Following this, the student learns about nutrition and digestion, the intake of food and its breakdown through pancreatic or hepatic enzymes, the uptake of lipids and proteins, the need for essential elements such as iodine, zinc, or iron, enterohepatic circulation, the important functions of the spleen, the function of gastric juices, the fragility of the gastric mucosal lining, and the functions of pancreatic juice and bile.

The students learn that life has been safeguarded for millions of years through ever-recurring processes, such as the uptake of oxygen from the tidal volume of air into the lungs and from there into the vascular pathways; the release of oxygen from the erythrocytes to the peripheral tissues; the excretion of urea, electrolytes, and water through the renal system; and the regulation of sodium and water at the macula densa of the kidneys. They will also be introduced to the important elementary building blocks of life: the sodium–water balance, the acid–base balance, calcium–magnesium metabolism, and the vital role of vitamins.

Hormones—the messengers of the body—account for the mode of action of the hypothalamic–pituitary axis. Hormones affect the pituitary gland, which in turn controls other glands (e.g., adrenal, thyroid, gonads). Epinephrine, norepinephrine, and tissue hormones make up the hormones of the sympathetic–adrenal medullary system.

The final topic of study for understanding the human body is the central nervous system and its functions, which the student has already become acquainted with during anatomy studies (**Fig. 3.3**). This final curricular unit involves knowledge about the body's reflexes and the transmission of stimuli from the peripheral to the central nervous system. The important functions of the cerebellum with regard to motor coordination, the basal ganglia, pain processing, the different pain fibers and the sensation of pain, and functions, such as language, consciousness, circadian rhythm, and the limbic system, are also part of this final unit. By the end of the physiology course, the student should understand the functions of each organ, the interaction of the organ groupings, and their fragility in the setting of a medical condition.

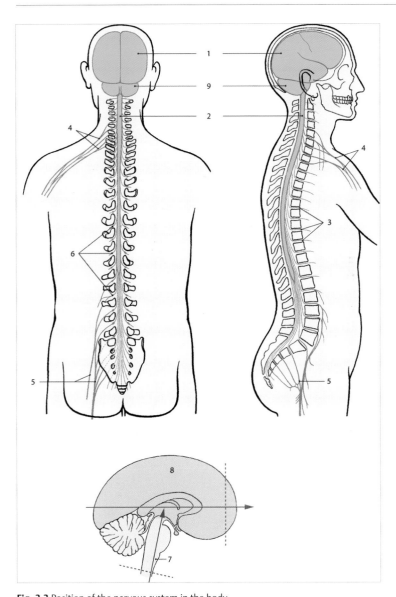

Fig. 3.3 Position of the nervous system in the body.
1 Encephalon, 2 Medulla spinalis, 3 Intervertebral foramina, 4 Brachial plexus, 5 Lumbosacral plexus, 6 Ganglia, 7 Brain stem, 8 Forebrain, 9 Cerebellum

The student will then learn about the structure of deoxyribonucleic acid (DNA), the metabolism of proteins and fatty acids, the hormonal mode of action, the basics of hepatic and renal biochemical functions, the connective and supportive tissues, and the muscles. The student will also become acquainted with the basics of biochemistry and the biochemical reactions in the body. It is worth mentioning that in some countries additional subjects, such as medical psychology, statistics, biomathematics, and cognitive sciences, are also taught. I have, however, focused on the fundamental subjects for this book. Having gained all of this knowledge, the student will now enter the next phase of medical studies, which addresses diseases in terms of general pathology, diagnostics, clinical examination, diagnostic radiology, and pharmacologic therapy.

A Quick Note

The student faces the enormous task of studying, memorizing, and capitalizing on all of this knowledge. Every physician has had to go through this. It can be done! Frustration or even capitulation is definitely not the way to go. Consistent studying and focusing on the subject alone will help the student understand medicine and learn and memorize important facts. However, as mentioned earlier in this section, our knowledge changes. Facts have a half-life, and the half-lives of medical knowledge are strikingly short. Soon after their state examination, young physicians may have forgotten most of what they learned in the areas of biochemistry and physiology. A surgeon, who is focused on knee and hip endoprosthetics, may have forgotten about the details of histology and embryology. The cardiologist who concentrates on cardiac arrhythmias may forget about the tendons in the ankle and the vascular tissue in the brain. This is a normal process that should not alarm or confuse anyone. However, it is crucial to learn and understand the overall context, that is, the basics of biochemistry, physiology, and human anatomy. Even after years or decades, one can read up on any subject, recapitulate what one has learned and find a new starting point with ease. The decisive factor when studying is to learn how to enthusiastically acquire knowledge and where to research things that have slipped from memory.

3.3 Pathology

The word *pathology* is derived from the Greek word *pathos*, which means "a passion" or "suffering," and from the Greek word *logos*, which can be translated as "teachings" or "word." The teaching of suffering and passion is one of the central pillars of medicine. Pathology is divided into macroscopic and microscopic sections, similar to the study of anatomy. Histopathology is further divided into cytology and the electromicroscopic and immunohistochemical depiction of tissues. Thus, pathology is the science of the abnormal processes of the human body.

Previously, students were introduced to the regular structure of the body macroscopically and microscopically in the anatomy section. Now, they will learn about pathologic changes, including malformation and inflammation or cell proliferation in the form of tumor tissue. Pathology also includes the origin of a disease, called the etiology, as well as the development and pathogenesis of disease. During the last few years, the fields of pathohistology, macroscopic pathology, pathobiochemistry, and pathophysiology have been on the rise. Pathobiochemistry explores the pathologic changes of metabolic processes and connective tissue, whereas pathophysiology is the study of the dilated heart and pathologically altered metabolic processes. Pathology forms the basis for describing organ and organ system diseases, as well as morbid, that is, pathological, syndromes.

Pathology and forensic medicine are strictly separated specialties. Forensic medicine, anatomy, and pathology are three specialties in which autopsies are performed. Forensic medicine is not primarily concerned with the pathologic changes of an organ or organ system, but instead with the clarification regarding the cause and the manner of death. A more in-depth review of forensic medicine will be included later on.

With regard to the study of pathology, students must learn two different things. First, they have to become acquainted with a great number of diseases and their corresponding microscopic and macroscopic changes. It is essential to have this armamentarium to master the clinical nomenclature. Similarly to other subjects, medical students must also *comprehend* the material and have a complete understanding of what the pathology describes. They must see a dilated heart, palpate it, and realize for themselves that this cardiac muscle cannot emit sufficient blood into the aorta. The medical student must learn that narrowing of the renal artery leads to high blood pressure. He or she must learn that the vascular supply of the intestines and the venous drainage into the liver indicate the filtering of tumor cells from the intestines into the liver. It is essential to gain an understanding of the pathologic changes in the individual organ systems, the pathologic functions of organs and organ systems, or syndromes that trigger diseases or are triggered by diseases that will cause further pathologic changes. Acquiring this understanding is, in addition to memorizing the malignancy stages of tumors, a vital part of pathology.

The aim of pathology is to recognize the origin and etiology of a particular disease so it can be diagnosed. The diagnosis is then followed by therapy, if available. In the case of available treatment, the patient may "*restitutio ad integrum*," or return to normal function. Therapy can also mean functional restrictions or limitations, as is the case in patients with myocardial disease. The adjuvants of pathology are the pathohistological study of histoid excisions, the collection of samples of histoid liquids (e.g., from the liver or osseous tissue from the iliac crest), and performing biopsy. Apart from the specification of the tissues and their further analysis, autopsy (derived from the Greek word *autopsia*, meaning "seeing for oneself") is one of the most important means of gathering insights into disease. Opening up the deceased person is often the only way to diagnose the disease.

Today's focus is on microscopic pathology (pathohistology) and macroscopic pathology (functional pathology). Neuropathology is another growing area of study involving the diagnosis of diseased tissues within the central nervous system. The core performance of histopathological diagnostics is the ability to diagnose neoplastic, inflammatory, and degenerative diseases with a high level of accuracy. Histopathological diagnosis is the basis for the assessment of tumors (benign/malignant), their specification and subspecification, prognostic assessment, and to determine the intensity of drug therapy and risk stratification. Defined stages are one of the means that aid histopathology by serving as the basis for classifying inflammatory diseases. Histopathology is an integral part of standard classification criteria, and it also plays an important role in infectious disease diagnostics due to the pathognomonic changes and the option of polymerase chain reaction (PCR) technology as a diagnostic tool. Because specific DNA amplicates via various sequencing and hybridization technologies, PCR-based technologies have become the foundation of molecular histopathological diagnostics.

Pathology also teaches us the principles of Rudolf Virchow, who, if you remember earlier in the chapter, taught us the idea that every cell originates from a cell (Virchow 1862). The student will start his or her learning in this subject on the topics of damage to and changes in cells, and will later learn about possible malformations (e.g., those caused by infections or fatty degeneration due to metabolic disorders). Students will then learn about cells and their functions, cell death, and the definition of necrosis. During autopsy and pathohistological examinations, the different forms of necrosis, such as enzymatic necrosis, gangrenous necrosis, necrosis of the extremities, and caseous necrosis in tuberculosis, will provide students with the first indications regarding a specific disease and its origin. Students taught pathology will also be introduced to the numerous types of possible noxious conditions that impact our bodies, including cold and heat (e.g., frostbites, burns), physical noxious agents, biologic noxious agents, and diseases caused by infections.

Next, the student learns about disorders of cell growth. The medical student must know how to differentiate metaplasia—the cell replacement of one type of tissue by another—from dysplasia, which is a reversible change, and from anaplasia, which is an irreversible change. The different types of tumors and tumor causes, the classification of malignancy levels and tumor stages, as well as highly specific tumor markers will deliver further indications about the course of disease. So, the student learns about tumors, their different stages, growth, proliferation, lymphatic regulation, their diffusion via venous drainage, metastasis, and malignancy, as well as classifying tumors into different stages. It is here that the student will learn about the tumor–node–metastasis staging system, a precise nomenclature that exists for all tumors in the human body, including benign and malignant tumors, and their proliferation and progression (**Fig. 3.4**). In the past, a tumor was surgically removed—a procedure that is critical for therapy. Today, however, in addition to surgery, chemotherapy, and radiotherapy, other methods for treating each specific tumor may be available. If applicable, radiotherapy may be the first step of treatment (e.g., in cases of rectal cancer), or the tumor may first be surgically removed and then followed up with radiotherapy (e.g., breast cancer). The new generation of chemotherapeutics and a variety of additional options will allow physicians to design an individual treatment plan for each tumor. The evaluation of the tumor, as well as other aspects of this entity (e.g., the immunohistochemical assessment of the genotype or the sensitivity in regard to pharmacotherapy), is the basis for deciding which treatment options to pursue.

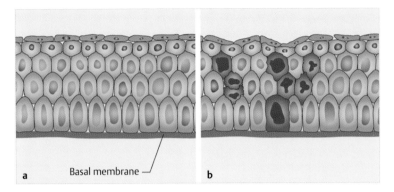

a   Basal membrane

b

Fig. 3.4 a–d Stages of tumor development.
a Normal squamous epithelium.
b Dysplasia: cellular and nuclear anomalies with cell layering retained.

Following the section on cell differentiation and cell growth, students will learn about the different types of inflammation according to their degree of complexity, progression, and proliferation. Students will then be able to ascertain diseases and their corresponding type of inflammation. For example, acute pancreatitis is an inflammation that inherently differs from a caseous granuloma in the setting of tuberculosis and one in the setting of superficial gastritis. Again, comprehension of the core material is essential for students to differentiate purulent inflammation from proliferating glomerular gastritis.

On that same point, let's look at clotting disorders. Clotting disorders, called hemorrhagic diatheses, present infrequently in general medicine. However, if they occur, their progression is often severe. Clotting disorders due to a lack of clotting factors can be difficult to control and complications can lead to fatal bleeding, particularly in women who are pregnant or patients undergoing surgery. Thromboses and embolisms are central complications in clotting disorders. Thus, it is important that students study the factors that can cause partial or complete vascular stenosis or vascular obstructions.

Students will also learn about diseases of the bone marrow and the blood. They will learn about zoonotic diseases, which occupy a central position in pathology. In addition, tumors of the male and female genitals cover another large section. Prostate and breast cancers are the most frequent carcinomas in males and females, respectively.

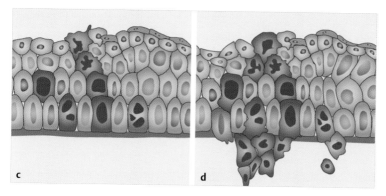

Fig. 3.4 a–d (continued) Stages of tumor development.
c Carcinoma in situ: cellular layering destroyed with basal membrane preserved.
d Invasive carcinoma: tumor cells have penetrated the basal membrane.

It is also important to recognize that pathology changes as scientific advancements are made. For example, students will learn about cardiac disorders, particularly cardiac hypertrophy, a coronary disease caused by the presence of arteriosclerotic plaques in the coronary arteries. As a person ages, vascular diseases come to the forefront. Research into early childhood cardiac disorders, including transposition of the aorta or the pulmonary trunk, have made it possible for these conditions to be surgically treated over the last few decades. Because of modern surgical advancements, infants with this condition may live 50 or 60 years. Thus, today's physicians see patients with disease that no physician ever saw in the past because advancements in science have given these patients longer survival rates. We must develop a sense of understanding for diseases and their morbid processes but also recognize the diversity of pathology.

3.4 Microbiology, Immunology, and Hygiene

Microbiology addresses the causes of diseases that have afflicted humans for thousands of years. Human history is often strongly impacted by great epidemics. Just think of the plague epidemics that befell the Roman Empire, or the Black Death that in medieval times killed millions of people. Think of the fast spread of syphilis in Europe. Some sources suggest that Columbus brought it back to Europe from his West Indies voyage. Military conflicts across Europe helped spread this venereal disease quickly and only with the discovery of penicillin was an effective cure found.

The history of the human race is also closely linked with the history of infections. The recognition of pathogenic microorganisms and their description were of particular importance. Only thereafter were drugs such as chemotherapeutics, antibiotics, and virostatic agents developed to fight specific microorganisms. The pasteurization of milk—a standard process in the food industry today—wound disinfection, and preventive vaccinations are rooted in microbiology and the successful works of people like Robert Koch. In 1876, Koch described the etiology of splenic fever (Koch 1876) and in 1882 the etiology of tuberculosis (Koch 1882, 1884). He travelled to distant countries to study disease; he explored malaria in Italy and New Guinea; his cholera expeditions to Egypt and India are legendary, earning him the Nobel Prize in 1905. Paul Ehrlich also delivered groundbreaking work in the areas of immunology and chemotherapy, as did Emil von Behring, Louis Pasteur, and others.

As in most other areas of medicine, classifications are needed in the field of microbiology so that we can recognize, diagnose, and treat various pathogens. Apart from identifying the special characteristics of bacteria, it is necessary for the medical student to learn about the basic and pathologic consequences of bacterial infection (**Fig. 3.5**). Some bacteria contain endotoxins in the cell wall while others produce exotoxins. There is a specific defense—that is, white blood cells release antibodies designed for specific proteins—and a nonspecific defense, which includes phagocytosis via tissue macrophages, the acidic pH value of the skin, as well as the stomach, salivary enzymes, and others. The virulence of a disease signifies the specific pathogenic triggers and the extent of such disease. An important aspect of microbiology is the exact transmission path of pathogens, whether it be through physical contact, via the air, or through contaminated water, among others.

The classification of microorganisms is based on the dyeability of the cell wall. This dye, the Gram stain, named after Hans Christian Gram, differentiates between gram-negative and gram-positive bacteria. Gram-negative bacteria have a monolayer peptidoglycan (murein) structure in which the dye does not create a lasting bond and can be washed out by alcohol. This destains the bacteria. Gram-positive bacteria have a multilayer peptidoglycan structure. The dye complexes build up within this structure and cannot be washed out with alcohol, so the bacteria turn the color blue. Bacteria are also differentiated into cocci, that is, spherical

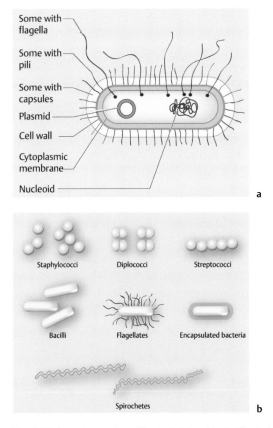

Some with flagella
Some with pili
Some with capsules
Plasmid
Cell wall
Cytoplasmic membrane
Nucleoid

a

Staphylococci   Diplococci   Streptococci

Bacilli   Flagellates   Encapsulated bacteria

Spirochetes   **b**

Fig. 3.5 Schematic structure of bacteria (**a**) and typical bacterial shapes (**b**).

bacteria, and bacilli, that is, rod-shaped bacteria. Gram-positive cocci include staphylococci, streptococci, and pneumococci. Gram-negative cocci include gonococci, the causative agent of gonorrhea, and meningococci, the causative agent of the much-feared meningitis. Gram-negative bacilli comprise a large group, including *Salmonella*, *Shigella*, *Yersinia*, and *Fusobacterium*. Aside from Gram stain, students will be introduced to other dye options, such as Ziehl–Neelsen stain, and Loeffler's methylene blue solution.

The classification of bacteria is essential, as is the description of the bacterium, the typical incubation period, possible complications, the ensuing infection, detection, and proof (be it microscopic, serologic, or even via animal experimentation), and the therapeutic options for treating the infection. In the context of microbiology, and later pharmacology, students are introduced to treatment resistance, particularly as it relates to antimicrobial therapy. Bacteria are able to exchange DNA—meaning they can share information—allowing them to develop resistance that can protect them against, for example, chemotherapeutics, which poses a problem that all hospitals must face. We encounter an increasing number of resistant strains that cause therapeutic ineffectiveness in high-performance medicines—similar to the days before the introduction of chemotherapeutics. Most physicians not involved in microbiology will eventually forget the different species of *Shigella* or the subtypes of endotoxins and exotoxins of individual groups of bacteria. However, the general understanding of microbiology, chemotherapy, and the increasing problem of resistance with unbounded dispensation of antibiotics is crucial. Chlamydia and fungal diseases are of special significance in, for example, immunodeficient patients following radiotherapy. It is important to remember that physicians must recognize the disease. They are only capable of doing so if they have thoroughly learned the basics of microbiology during the course of their studies. They can look up later what they do not remember.

Immunology addresses the defense system of the body. Here, we differentiate between the specific and the nonspecific systems. Nonspecific defense consists of different types of cells such as macrophages in the tissue and those in the blood stream. With regard to specific defense, we differentiate between B and T lymphocytes expressed after contact with an antigen in order to work as a tissue protein for the specific defense (**Fig. 3.6**). Various disease groups are based on allergic reactions; hypersensitivity reactions caused by antibodies or T lymphocytes. They are rare but nonetheless arise suddenly and with severity.

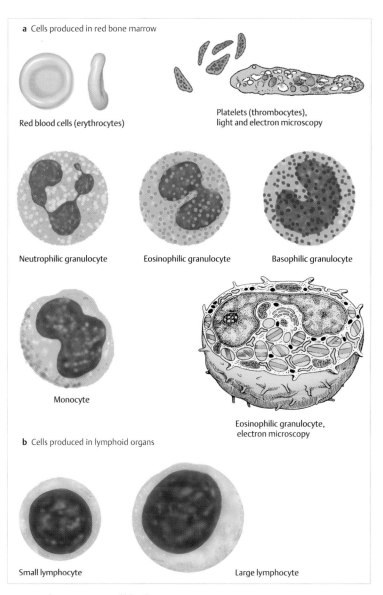

Fig. 3.6 a,b Components of blood.

In 1928, Alexander Fleming discovered the antibacterial properties of penicillin when he examined the effects of the chance encounter between a staphylococci colony and a mold fungus. He laid the foundation for the beginnings of antibacterial therapy. However, the increasing bacterial resistance we see today is partly due to the frequency with which farm animals receive high doses of antibiotics before they are slaughtered for food. In some countries, this may be the only way to keep the meat supply steady. But what is the price? The development of antibiotic-resistant germs forms a vicious cycle. The development of drug resistance among bacteria seen in the intensive care setting is the latest proof of the detrimental outcome of uncontrolled antibiotic administration.

Edward Jenner discovered that humans could be protected from smallpox by receiving a vaccination with cowpox. This therapy called vaccination, derived from the Latin word vacca for "cow," used the inoculation of bacteria or viruses or their components, thereby proving that we are not helplessly subjected to infection. Some great physicians were daring and determined enough to help humankind. It was sensational at the time that Edward Jenner infected his own children to prove his theory. The people of his hometown and the medical community were solidly against him and tried to revoke the license of this supposed quack. Nevertheless, Edward Jenner is an example for the currently unsolvable problems of our times in infection diseases.

In the broadest sense, hygiene covers all aspects of health maintenance, including the prevention of human diseases or disease-causing behavior. Hygiene is undoubtedly useful and necessary. Still, the physician-to-be may occasionally ask themselves about the necessity of discussing the bacterial count in drinking water or the intensity of lights in the workplace. The field of hygiene is large and many of its aspects are taken for granted in Western societies. Drinkable water is an example of this mindset. We only have to go to Mexico, however, to find out that regular tap water is not potable, or that we cannot conduct daily dental hygiene with regular tap water because it contains an excessive amount of germs unknown to our intestines and will cause illness if ingested. *Salmonella* or *Shigella* outbreaks in Western Europe provoked by frozen strawberries or beans from China delivered to commercial kitchens could be devastating. Produce contaminated in China does not undergo the same vigorous controls that are standard in Western European and North American countries. Comparable situations occur on cruise ships where the norovirus has infected thousands of passengers and staff.

It could be said that an implicit attitude to hygiene is standard and so we need not make particular mention of it. This applies to personal hygiene, such as taking regular showers, brushing one's teeth daily, and caring for one's hair and genitals. However, although people in Western European and North American countries adhere to these hygienic standards, the World Health Organization says that many people in Third World countries cannot do so because of the lack of water. Hygiene also applies to our living space and includes psychological hygiene. Relaxation in the tenements of big cities is often impossible. Stress, noise from neighbors, the impossibility of opening a window because of the traffic below, and perpetually bright lighting are factors that turn the living space into an irritant that can cause disease.

We are told that healthy nutrition (another branch of hygiene) means having a balanced mixed diet, which, for some, may include consuming fish once or twice a week. If the global population ate fish only once a week, there would be no more fish in the world's oceans after 6 months. We are facing difficult challenges that are, logistically speaking, difficult or nearly impossible to solve. Part of this difficulty is in supplying the global population with adequate food. In Western countries, we increasingly focus on healthy nutrition. Healthy nutrition is only "healthy" if we know where our food comes from. Unintentional poisonings due to pesticides or heavy metals are on the decline at the same time as epidemic infections with bacteria and viral diseases are on the rise.

These frequently theoretic and dry-sounding subjects are important for the understanding of medicine, and every physician should master their basics.

3.5 Patient History and Examination

Every treatment begins with the medical consultation. Except in cases of emergency, the interaction between the physician and patient is the foundation of every treatment.

When a patient seeks a physician for advice, information, or help regarding a disorder or impairment, the ensuing conversation must be carried out with great sensitivity, particularly at the onset. Fritz Meerwein (1969) succinctly summarized the relevant aspects of the initial clinical interview:

- What concern does the patient present with today?
- How do they present their concern?
- Why do they present it that way?
- What do they present unknowingly?
- Why have they presented it to me?
- Has the patient accepted my diagnosis and therapy plan?

Every physician should pose these questions to help develop the sensibility to properly respond to the patient. Friedrich Schettler (1985) recommends beginning the physician–patient interaction with questions regarding the causes that brought the patient to see the physician. Physicians should allow the patient to report while listening and observing without interjecting. In so doing, the physicians first orient themselves and assess their approach. If possible, they ask pointed questions to narrow the diagnosis. Disapproving gestures, shoulder shrugging, head shaking, or snide remarks with regard to previous treatment are not appropriate. This includes the fact that demeanor, restrained gestures, and appropriate clothing are crucial attributes of a physician. Whether at the doctor's office, walk-in clinic, or the hospital, the patient is in a highly delicate situation. The disease, ailment, or questions are often located very close to his or her "self." They are looking for advice, for the aid of the physician, because they are unable to handle the symptoms that unsettle them.

Patients provide plenty of nonverbal information. It is well worth paying attention to the way they enter the doctor's office, sit in their hospital room, or lie in bed. Are they approachable, do they look at the physician, is their face contorted with pain or relaxed, are they focused on the conversation with the physician, are they absent-minded, are they euphoric or depressed? All this information is important for the physician to get the right start to the conversation and properly respond to the patient. Ultimately, the patient is looking for advice and help from the physician, not the other way around. The physician's opening question is essential. Frequently, physicians begin the consultation with a question, such as "What can I do for you?" or "What brings you here?" One could also ask, "What is your ailment?" or "How can I help you?" Sometimes doctors view the latter as emphasizing the "serving" aspect of the physician's role too much. Beginning the consultation with the question, "What is your ailment?" can lead to a defensive attitude in some patients. In his *Textbook of Psychiatry*, the Swiss psychiatrist Paul Eugen Bleuler (1983) summarized this everyday situation:

Facing the great task to help a patient, the physician has two options:

1. He can observe the ailment. He can then conclude one of the disease patterns from the disease symptoms. This will tell him the available treatment methods from which he will select and apply the proper ones for his patient.
2. He can also choose another path: he can listen to the patient like a familiar friend. That makes him shift part of his attention from diagnosing an ailment, noting psychopathological symptoms and rendering an impersonal diagnosis to appreciating a person in their uniqueness and sharing their hardships, fears, wishes, and expectations.

It is vital that the patient confides in the physician and is willing to share a common path, and have the physician diagnose and later treat the ailment. The physician should be impartial and take the time to truly listen and understand what the patient thinks and how they express themselves. This way the physician can give them the best possible individualized care. The physician can give the patient a personalized response and communicate his understanding and ability to help.

The differentiation between being sick and the disease is more precise in the English language than it is in German, for example. The term *disease* denotes the medical description and definition of the respective ailment. The term *illness* denotes the perspectives of the patient and includes the feelings and experiences of the patient about the ailment. There is a third term, *sickness*, which denotes the external perspective of the patient's friends and family about the condition and its effect on society.

It is self-evident that during the physician–patient consultation the physician devotes all of his or her attention and time to the patient and must not be interrupted by the phone or medical colleagues or by anything else. Patients often feel positively toward the physician if he or she takes them seriously and is responsive to them. Patients must feel that the physician is willing to perceive and recognize their problems. They must not feel that they are in some sort of repair shop for organic symptoms. It is necessary to point out that this requires the cooperation of the patient. In this context, physician and medical historian Hans Schadewaldt (1964) describes the view of the physician and patient role in ancient times:

It was essential that sick people consulted the physician in time. What is so special and unique to us regarding the ancient view is that the physician was not supposed to address the disease immediately. According to Hippocrates he had to convince the patient to cooperate. If the person was not willing or able to cooperate every reputable physician was supposed to decline treatment.

In essence, the patient was supposed to be encouraged to actively participate so that both the physician and patient could discern the correct diagnosis and treatment.

The patient must be willing to talk about his or her ailment and the physician must be willing to hear what is said. For example, the subject of obesity should be addressed with a patient who is overweight, as well as any bad habits or unhealthy diet. The same applies to someone who smokes—the physician should discuss the damaging effects of smoking with them. Mere diagnosis and treatment of the disease, for example, a circulatory disorder of the leg with subsequent vascular surgery, are insufficient if smoking goes unaddressed. The patient must learn what leads to the symptoms of disease; this knowledge is crucial to lifestyle changes. This implies that the physician must be willing to listen and possess the willingness and competence to bring up unpleasant issues regarding necessary lifestyle changes. This includes the necessity of insisting that the patient at least *considers* these changes. In the long term, simply treating disease without recognizing further consequences will not help the patient. A confused patient with a circulatory disorder in the brain due to arteriosclerotic vascular changes requires treatment. If this patient receives a laceration to the head due to a fall, then wound treatment is required, but, ultimately, this treatment alone is insufficient. The underlying disease must be treated and then the patient must be advised to take precautions to avoid future injuries. To truly treat the disease, it is the aim of the medical consultation to create awareness and understanding in the patient, to communicate the origin of certain symptoms, and explain why certain changes in the body have taken place.

In addition, an informative consultation regarding surgery must clarify the risks and benefits. The patient may want to know why he or she is sick and what must be done to eliminate or alleviate the disease. This surgical consultation includes explaining the disease, pointing out the effects of the disease, benefits and risks of surgery, and likelihood of survival. The patient should come to a careful and considered decision as to whether to undergo surgery. The physician should explain to the patient what caused the disorder and how to best and most efficiently treat this condition. It is insufficient—and above all is not expedient—to tell them that surgery is the best choice, or vaunt one's own medical competence, or have the patient fill out a patient consent form, sign it, and thank them for their time and attention. The patient must be informed of all the information relevant to their condition, otherwise they cannot come to an informed decision and cannot, therefore, truly provide consent for treatment. The patient has the right to learn about their condition and what measures could and should be taken to help their individual situation. Ultimately, the patient has the right to terminate or shorten the relationship. Here, too, the physician should attune themselves to the patient.

Frequently, communication between the physician and older people, children, people whose first language or cultural practices are different from that of the physician, patients with cancer, or those who are terminally ill, may be emotionally charged. For example, with an older person, the physician might want to devote more time to the visit, explaining the facts in ways appropriate for and relevant to the patient so that they can understand what the physician is saying and make informed choices. The physician may have to repeat what he or she has already stated. It is true that some older patients will indicate that they understand the explanations of the physician, but do not remember the conversation the next day. With children, a different type of language is required, and their parents must also be involved in the conversation. Physicians must take pediatric patients and their concerns seriously. They should be addressed neither with "baby talk" nor in a professional language that can intimidate them. Patients with cancer may recognize the limits of modern-day medicine and may want to know the whole truth from the physician—or not. In this case, physicians should impart their knowledge cautiously, providing all relevant medical knowledge to the patient based on the needs and preferences of the patient. Of course, it is rare for anyone to want to hear—even if they say they do—that they have a tumor and are likely to live only for a short time. The physician must possess the sensitivity to respond to the patient adequately and explain the available diagnostic or therapeutic measures and help the patient determine an appropriate management option based on the patient's needs and preferences. Karl Jaspers 1958 summarized it as follows: "The patient does not really want to know b2ut obey. The authority of the physician is a desirable fixed position, which relieves him of his deliberations and responsibility. The more severe the patient's disease the greater is his willingness to follow the physician." Karl Jaspers is certainly right that the physician is an authority and a wished-for point of reference that the patient commits to or even latches on to. However, the physician should exchange views with the patient about his or her individual situation.

The patient's thoughts about their disease, their expectations, fears, wishes, and hopes all factor into the course of the disease. Thus, we need only disclose the information we judge to be medically relevant to the patient, but we must do so in a respectful and sensitive manner, tailoring the information we provide to meet the needs and preferences of our patients. Not using therapeutic privilege, or misgauging what our patients need and want could be disastrous. However, in general, one cannot use medical authority to put the patient off until later, to avoid telling them the truth, and to leave them uninformed. After all, the physician is not only aware of his or her own abilities but also of the medical futility of treatment in a patient with advanced-stage cancer, but what should the physician say? What should he or she not say? What is the limit and where is confidence betrayed? It is crucial that the physician is willing to attune themselves to the patient's needs and desires. The medical consultation cannot turn into an interrogation or question-and-answer session. The dialog must be free of constraints and the roles clearly defined. The physician is the authority and in spite of all the leveling down, the physician's demeanor during the medical consultation is decisive. In my experience, the patient presents because they see the physician as a medical expert. The basic attitude conveyed by the physician should be earnest but cheerful and willing to respond to the patient. The question "There is nothing wrong with you, what are you doing here?" has no place in a physician's consultation.

It is also inappropriate for the physician to treat the patient as if they were an entity or a number. Some authors report that physicians are allowed 3 minutes for each consultation and frequently multitask during the conversation. According to German physician Linus S. Geisler (2002), a resident physician may spend 60% to 80%—and the hospital physician up to 50%—of his or her working time on patient consultation. Communication appears to be insignificant when measured against the impressive potential of today's medicine. Other authors report that 7 to 8 minutes are allowed for each physician–patient consultation. No matter how much time is spent in reality, the effect on the patient and whether or not the physician is helpful is what makes the difference.

In addition to their trust in the physician, the patient must trust in something else—the *therapy*. The positive effects of some drugs are beyond question, but it is astounding to see how placebos can improve or alleviate symptoms—sometimes in as many as 40% of patients for some conditions. Medication cost is another important factor regarding patient adherence. The physician can foster the self-healing power of the patient if the patient believes in the physician and trusts them and if the physician can give direction to the patient. Even if they are apt, negative remarks about colleagues in the presence of a patient, comments that one would have done this or that differently, or that a treatment was uncalled for, may unnerve the patient.

In this context, the Milgram experiment must be mentioned (Milgram 1974). This experiment is about obedience and human behavior. Actions executed at command and those executed voluntarily fundamentally differ. A simple experiment teaches us about the willingness to obey. The volunteer enters a laboratory and receives the order to witness a series of activities. These activities are likely to cause increasing moral conflict in the volunteer. The central question is: How long will the volunteer obey the directive of the examiner before he refuses to follow orders? The volunteer watches a student being strapped to a shock generator. The student is connected to the shock generator, which can emit electric shocks between 15 and 450 volt. The volunteer does not know that the generator is a dummy. The involved teacher and student are privy to the set up and play their rolls. The teacher asks a question. The student answers the question. The teacher punishes the student with an electric shock if the answer is wrong. This punishment by itself is ethically unacceptable. Thus, every volunteer watching this series of experiments should immediately abort the test because punishment through electric shock is unacceptable in our society. How far will the volunteer go? In general, the student pretended to display discomfort at 75 V. At 150 V, he asked to terminate the experiment. At 285 V the student blurted out inarticulate shouts of pain. Step by step, the volunteer is led further into moral conflict. The moment he hesitated to continue or was ready to abort the test, he received the order to continue. Most volunteers yielded. The reluctance to break with authority was huge.

I mention the Milgram experiment to highlight the idea of authority and its dynamics. Today, it is frowned upon in certain circles to speak of authority or authority figures but the concept certainly deserves to be discussed. On the one hand we cannot negate the existing respect for authority. On the other hand, patients "consent," not "obey," so authority in the old sense is not appropriate in the physician–patient relationship. The patient is looking for advice. The capacity of the physician–patient relationship becomes apparent especially in difficult situations.

We demand much from physicians. They must accept the patient as an equal and tell them the truth, but in medical diagnostics, the truth is often brutal. The physician may feel they cannot always tell the entire truth, but must communicate what they think is appropriate. It cannot be stressed enough how important informed consent is, and that all relevant medical information has to be disclosed to patients. But physicians may use their judgment in how to do this and meet the individual patients' needs at the same time. The way in which they explain the truth can vary, for example, using layperson's terms, but they have to obtain truly informed consent from a patient to start or end treatment. Counseling techniques can be learned. Bioethics, bedside manner, and counseling are all topics taught in medical schools today and can help the physician better connect and communicate with the patient. Ultimately, physicians should simply try to be themselves—human beings who want to help.

3.6 Pharmacology

Treatment recommendations, guidelines, and drug approval vary among the various regions. What is presented here may not be specific to the individual reader's country. More detailed information can be obtained from official sources, for example, the Food and Drug Administration (FDA) in the United States, the National Institute for Health and Care Excellence (NICE) in the UK and the Federal Institute for Drugs and Medical Devices (Bundesinstitut für Arzneimittel und Medizinprodukte, BfArM) in Germany.

Generally speaking, pharmacology is about substances. The body is supplied with these substances (e.g., synthesized substances, plant compounds). This can be done intravenously, via the skin or gastrointestinal tract, or through inhalation, among other methods. The substances spread inside the body and are then eliminated again. They may be excreted through the kidneys or bile, or they may be metabolized in the liver. The substances are administered in certain doses and time intervals for the purpose of diagnostics or treatment.

The medicinal product is the pharmaceutical preparation of the drug substance. Efficiently administered in this way, it can affect or explore the physiologic system or the pathologic condition of the patient. A great variety of systemic applications are available (e.g., oral, intravenous, intra-arterial, intrathecal, percutaneous). The choice depends on the resorption rate and bioavailability of the medicinal substance and their dependence on the type of application. Additional medicinal substances primarily focus on a nonsystemic local effect (e.g., powders, salves, or hydrogels used in dermatology).

The research and development of new medicinal substances and products are demanding and time consuming. Consequently, these methods are costly and strictly guided by economic considerations, sometimes leading to medicinal oversupply for frequently encountered diseases, or a shortage of adequate drugs for rare diseases. In general, the development of new drugs specifically used to target diseases common in financially weak Third World countries is also scarce.

The challenge in selecting the proper medicinal substances and products is complicated in the Western world by the fact that the same substance is also offered in different forms by different producers and can eventually be marketed as a trade-name drug. In addition to that, many so-called "new" developments offer only slight changes to already existing therapeutic concepts. They do not always offer improvement and are called "me too" drugs.

Once chosen, the next demanding challenge is properly applying the preferred drug. To ensure the safe and effective administration of medicinal substances, knowledge about numerous aspects regarding the substances is required, including their pharmacologic properties, intake efficiency, distribution in the body, pathways and duration of their elimination from the body, possible formation of pharmacologically effectual metabolites, interaction with other drugs, as well as knowledge about age-, sex-, or disease-specific changes of the above characteristics.

Paracelsus' (1538) famous quotation, *"Dosis sola venenum facit"*, meaning, literally "The dose alone makes the poison" holds true. This is why students are first introduced to general pharmacology and later to its more specific aspects. It is important to understand the principles of the dose-and-effect relationship. These principles relate to the nominal dose and the amount of the medicinal substance reaching its target location and receptors.

Pharmaceuticals can often have no effect if they are given in inadequate doses. An excessive dose can damage the body. The best drug cannot work without being absorbed by the body. In this context, the understanding of receptor theory is essential. A receptor is like a negative imprint of a drug that enables a bond to form between it and the drug, thus triggering the intracellular effect. If they are given in too high a dose, drugs entering the placenta of a pregnant woman may put the embryo or fetus at risk. Here, knowledge of drugs and the body's interactions are vital.

Most textbooks about pharmacology begin with parasympathomimetics as antidotes in cases of intoxication and parasympatholytics in cases of intestinal spasm. In physiology, we were introduced to the parasympathetic and sympathetic nervous systems. The modular concept of medical studies is continued in pharmacology. Within the group of sympathomimetics and sympatholytics we will take a closer look at medications used for high blood pressure and hypertension.

Over the years, pharmaceuticals in cardiology have changed significantly. Digitalis compounds are being replaced more and more by β-blockers and angiotensin-converting enzyme (ACE) inhibitors. Coronary dilators are still of high value, especially in cases of angina pectoris. Acute myocardial infarction and hypertensive crisis are primarily treated pharmacologically. Nitro compounds, heparin, oxygen, β-blockers, and aspirin are the substances primarily administered during myocardial infarctions. Every physician must know the pharmacology for renal diseases, especially for diuretic disorders and imbalances in sodium and potassium levels.

With regard to the gastrointestinal tract, the era of ulcer surgery has belonged to the past ever since the introduction of proton pump inhibitors. Emphasis is placed on emetics, antiemetics, and the treatment of Crohn's disease. In the era of metabolic diseases, focus is placed on gout medication, called uricosuric and uricostatic drugs, carbohydrate metabolism, and insulin, or insulin analogs in cases of diabetes mellitus.

The student learns about another main area of pharmacology composed of antibiotic treatments, including penicillin, cephalosporin, sulfonamides, and antimitotics. Increasing bacterial resistance continues to pose problems to the pharmacologic medicine of the twenty-first century. We are approaching conditions similar to those prior to World War II when pharmacologic treatment for infections did not yet exist, although there have been recent breakthroughs in antibiotics—considered by some to be "game changers" (Wright 2015). Today, we have many choices of antibiotics, but some bacteria have become resistant to these drugs, which then produce no antibiotic effect.

The vast area of chemotherapy for use in oncology is gaining significance, as is the treatment of poisoning, which has become a focal point of pharmacology. Mainly in Western countries, the number of poisonings with arsenic, lead, chrome, other heavy metals, and insecticides has decreased. However, particularly in the urban Western world, intoxication with alcohol and synthetic drugs, such as heroin, cocaine, lysergic acid diethylamide (commonly known as LSD) and the like, is on the rise.

In the area of internal diseases, focus is placed on hormones, hormonal treatment of thyroid disorders, contraceptive treatment, treatment with adrenal hormones, and the use of calcitonin.

Neuropharmacology requires particular consideration. Patient compliance is crucial. We will learn later, in the section on psychiatry, about reaching one's own therapeutic limits as a physician. For instance, a patient with schizophrenia is treated with the neuroleptic haloperidol and experiences symptom improvement. After a latency period of 6 or 12 months, the patient may decide to discontinue the drug because they believe they now feel healthy, and they then slip into a psychotic crisis. Often, the patient may not even realize this relapse. This is a compliance problem that can occur with patients prescribed psychotropic drugs. In general, psychotropic drugs must be individually dosed.

Although they were previously prescribed as sleeping aids, barbiturates, also called hypnotics, interfere with the sleeping rhythm and suppress neuronal activity in the reticular formation. Due to the inhibiting effect on the respiratory center, they are also abused, in cases of suicide, for example.

We will closely study Parkinson's disease in the neurology unit, a disorder marked by an absolute and relative deficiency of dopamine in the central nervous system. Levodopa remains the gold standard for the treatment of patients with Parkinson's disease based on the dopamine deficiency in the substantia nigra. Adverse events of levodopa use include allergic reactions, bone marrow damage, and the intensification of angle-closure glaucoma with raised intraocular pressure. Additional active substances that can be used for Parkinson's disease include dopamine antagonists, such as ropinirole, bromocriptine, apomorphine, rotigotine, and pramipexole, monoamine oxidase B (MAO-B) inhibitors (e.g., selegiline), anticholinergics, and others. The drug amantadine is also used in

Parkinson's disease, but less for rigor than for tremor and akinesia. Preferably, patients receive therapy at specialized centers offering individually customized medical care, pharmacologic treatment, and physical and occupational therapy. Side effects are a determining factor, especially in Parkinson's disease. Frequently in older patients, a medication prescribed to help alleviate the symptoms of the disease must be discontinued because of the side effects of the drug. This is a very frustrating situation for both the patient and the physician.

Antidepressants constitute another large group of neuropharmaceuticals. They are prescribed for states of depression, anxiety, and stress disorders. Tricyclic antidepressants inhibit the reuptake of norepinephrine and serotonin in the synaptic cleft. Thus, the catecholamine concentration is increased in the cleft, allowing the catecholamines an extended effect. Undesired adverse events of tricyclic antidepressants can include constipation, voiding disorders, tachycardia, mouth dryness, and elevated intraocular pressure. The latter can cause irreversible damage in patients with glaucoma. Consideration must also be given to the fact that during the initial phase of taking these drugs, the inner drive increases while suicidal notions remain. Attempted suicides must be prevented by concurrently giving benzodiazepine. Monoamine oxidase inhibitors (MAOIs) constitute the second-largest group of antidepressants. In recent years, considerable changes have also taken place within this group of drugs. Today, we differentiate between nonselective and irreversible monoamine oxidase inhibitors. The latter causes increased neurotransmitter concentration by inhibiting monoamine oxidase. It is vital to instruct the patient that he or she must not simultaneously consume tyramine, or a hypertensive crisis may result. One type of food containing tyramine is cheese. (This is a very popular pharmacology exam question!) Other antidepressants include the following:

- Selective serotonin reuptake inhibitors (SSRIs), such as fluoxetine and paroxetine, which inhibit the selective reuptake of serotonin.
- The selective norepinephrine reuptake inhibitor (NRI) reboxetine.
- Dual selective serotonin and norepinephrine reuptake inhibitors (SNRIs).

Ultimately, they all cause an elevated concentration of transmitters at the synaptic cleft as a means to treat depressive states.

The next group of psychotropic drugs contains mood tranquilizers, including lithium, valproic acid, and carbamazepine. In particular, lithium has a very narrow therapeutic index. Blood must be regularly taken during the intake of this substance. In the event of a lithium overdose, seizures, ataxias, or cardiac arrhythmias may occur.

Neuroleptics constitute the next large group of neuropharmaceuticals. They are still the gold standard of treatment for schizophrenia. Neuroleptics have a cushioning effect in hallucinations, delusions, and compulsive ideas. They reduce inner drive and tension. These types of drugs include the following:

- Phenothiazine derivatives (promethazine and triflupromazine).
- Butyrophenone derivatives (e.g., haloperidol).
- Dibenzodiazepines (e.g., clozapine).

The necessity for administering these drugs in the event of hallucinations, delusions, and compulsive ideas is not to deny their undesired adverse events, which can include tremor, dyskinesias, cardiac complications, hormonal changes, skin alterations, increased photosensitivity, and, specific to clozapine, agranulocytosis.

The final group of psychotropic drugs I would like to mention is anxiolytics. In contrast to other drugs, the way anxiolytics work in the system has been largely resolved. Benzodiazepines form a specific bond with the benzodiazepine receptor of the γ-aminobutyric acid (GABA) receptor and changes the conformation. The alteration of the receptor causes an opening of the chloride ion channels in the neuron membrane, which in turn causes the cell to be less excitable. The typical effects of benzodiazepine use include reduced anxiety, muscle relaxation, and sedation. Thus, frequently they are used for patients with anxiety, tension, restlessness, and sleeping disorders. Diazepam is a choice in cases of epilepsy. Due to its broad therapeutic index, it is unlikely that intoxication will occur.

Some hospitals in the Western world have begun to employ their own pharmaceutical drug commissions and pharmacologists. The control and execution of an expansive clinical study and concurrent treatment of patients are almost mutually exclusive. Contributing factors to this situation are the resistance development of antibiotics mentioned above and the increasing complexity of clinical studies regarding therapeutic improvement. Pharmacologists in the United States, for example, should confirm that the hospital and its staff comply with the Clinical Laboratory Improvement Amendments regulations. Some hospitals have begun to employ additional pharmacologists to address questions and issues relating to such topics as allergic reactions, heparin use, drug interactions, and the use of pharmaceuticals in aging patients.

Pharmacology is the foundation of internal medicine, and it is a demanding field that is subjected to constant changes and is likely to remain one of the most essential disciplines of medicine.

3.7 Radiology

In 1895, Wilhelm Conrad Roentgen published his paper, "On a new kind of rays", which was the beginning of X-ray diagnostics. Today, we cannot conceive of medicine without it. Radiology comprises the three large areas of X-ray diagnostics, nuclear medicine, and radiotherapy (**Fig. 3.7**).

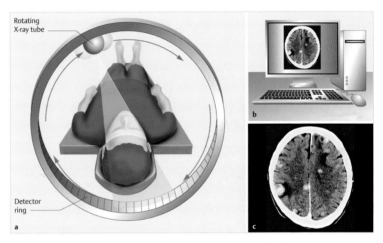

Fig. 3.7 (a–c) The principle of X-ray computed tomography (CT). The example shows cranial CT in a patient with brain metastases.

Radiology education generally builds on the knowledge the student gained during medical physics, which is typically taught during preclinical studies. There is a growing understanding in our society regarding the importance of radiation protection. It is vital that the physician-to-be understands the actual and potential damage of nuclear radiation. In particular, gonadal DNA damage is a good example of the danger of high-energy rays. This damage is irreversible and can be passed on for generations. Radiation with kinetic energy at levels higher than 5 eV can ionize and cause genetic damage. Unfortunately, we cannot yet abandon the use of ionizing radiation in radiation oncology, nuclear medicine, or in diagnostic radiology.

However, considerable change has taken place in diagnostic radiology in the past years. Fluoroscopic examinations using contrast agents were abandoned in the area of the esophagus, stomach, and the intestines and instead have been replaced by endoscopic procedures. Alternative procedures, such as capsule endoscopy in intestinal diagnostics, are currently being re-evaluated. Traditional X-ray diagnostics are still obtained, particularly of the lungs and the skeleton. In addition to the ability to diagnose pulmonary disease, conventional X-rays can also provide important information about the size and function of the heart and vessels. This type of imaging study is cost effective, quick, and can be obtained using a low exposure to radiation. The same holds true for skeletal survey radiography, which is still the preferred imaging method in traumatology (**Fig. 3.8**).

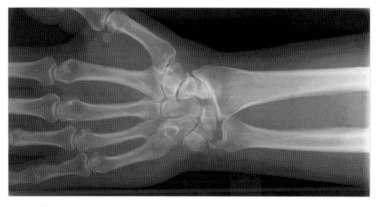

Fig. 3.8 X-ray of the hand showing scapholunate advanced collapse stage III.

A later addition to imaging methods is ultrasonography, which has superseded many conventional areas of X-ray diagnostics, particularly in differential diagnoses of the large organs of the upper abdomen (pancreas, liver, kidneys, spleen). For example, interventional radiology of the heart via ionizing radiation has lost its significance. Angiography of the vessels can frequently be replaced by magnetic resonance imaging (MRI) and computed tomography (CT). In fact, the use of MRI revolutionized the entire field of sectional imaging in the 1980s.

Interventional therapeutic measures frequently replace surgery; for example, CT-guided biopsies to collect tissue samples. Balloon dilatation and stent implantation are examples of the use of radiology, particularly for use in coronary arteries and as treatment options for stenosis or circulatory disorders of the large vessels. Relatively new to the field is radiologic intervention in the event of liver metastasis using radiofrequency ablation or selective internal radiation therapy (SIRT), which is conducted in collaboration with nuclear medicine specialists. During this method, microspheres are placed inside the tumor vessels, with the aim of sealing them and cutting the tumor off from its source of nutrition.

Transarterial chemoembolization (TACE) is a procedure in which chemotherapeutic substances are administered directly into the tumor via radiologically inserted catheters. Side effects from the procedure can be reduced due to the quasilocal nature of this treatment. Although it is still in its experimental stage, nanotherapy has been used as an effective interventional treatment for liver metastases. During this procedure, liquid ferric particles are docked onto chemotherapeutic agents and intravenously administered to the patient; however, this is a salvage or palliative therapeutic measure. The liquid ferric particles possess a high affinity for the mononuclear phagocyte system of the liver; consequently, high concentrations of the conjugate are found in this area. This is another type of quasilocal chemotherapy.

The field of diagnostic nuclear medicine has also drastically changed in recent years. In the past, nuclear medicine traditionally dealt with in vivo diagnostics, such as bone, thyroid, and kidney sequence scintigraphy, and the treatment of benign or malignant thyroid disorders. Today, nuclear medicine has shifted in the direction of sectional imaging diagnostic methods such as single photon emission–computed tomography (SPECT) or positron emission tomography–computed tomography (PET-CT). PET is a whole-body sectional imaging method that displays morphologic structures and metabolic processes. It is performed via the intravenous administration of radioactively marked substances. PET-CT has become a valuable diagnostic tool in tumor diseases and brain function testing. The treatment of benign or malignant thyroid diseases remains a central focus in nuclear medicine.

Radiotherapy, also called radio-oncology, is an interesting specialty that involves most areas of medicine. Therapy begins with an individually designed treatment plan. Tumors in places such as the prostate or head and neck are displayed, analyzed, and the adequate ray intensity is calculated by way of three-dimensional conformal or intensity-modulated radiotherapy. In most areas of oncology, general treatment plans for tumors are outdated. In modern times, tumors are staged in terms of their size and dimension and are systematically treated according to applicable guidelines. Scientists compile these evidence-based guidelines partly on the findings of randomized trials. These guidelines generally result in recommendations of therapeutic options for various oncologic diseases, thus leading to a quantitative shift in the use of the three therapeutic pillars (surgery, radiotherapy, and chemotherapy). Combination treatments—in particular, radiotherapy/chemotherapy—frequently avoid the need for surgery, for example, in some cases of anal cancer, certain types of esophageal cancer, most head and neck tumors, and many types of lung cancer. New procedures in this area include: (1) stereotactic radiation therapy of the central nervous system and other areas of the body, where a targeted radiation beam destroys the tumor during a few sessions; (2) single-dose stereotaxis, also called radiosurgery, in which the tumor is cauterized instead of cut during a single session using highly collimated rays.

For cases of prostate cancer, brachytherapy has been available for some time. Particularly in the early stages of prostate cancer, brachytherapy produces better outcomes than surgery or percutaneous irradiation without serious adverse events. The field of radio-oncology is constantly changing as technical developments during the last 20 years have followed in quick succession.

Proton therapy is currently experiencing a revival. It irradiates the tumor and is accurate to the millimeter; it provides only minimal exposure to the surrounding healthy tissue. This therapy is useful for pediatric tumors and in tumors of the central nervous system.

3.8 Internal Medicine

Internal medicine is one of the core subjects of medicine. It covers the internal diseases of a human being. In the past, neurology and laboratory medicine were also part of this specialty. In previous eras, medical professors would also teach pharmacology as part of internal medicine. The therapeutic approach in internal medicine used to be conservative drug therapy. In modern times, interventional procedures, such as stent implantation in constricted coronary vessels or endoscopic polyp or tumor ablation, are gaining importance. This importance also applies to clinical practice and education.

We can diagnose and treat growing numbers of diseases due to the wealth of knowledge acquired through medical research and scientific advancement. The use of more precise diagnostic methods, such as CT and MRI, allows us to increase the speed and accuracy with which we can view the body. Newer-generation sonographic units produce excellent high-definition images (**Fig. 3.9**). Used by an experienced physician, they can deliver valuable noninvasive insights into disease processes. Therapies for many diseases are subject to constant change. For example, the latest generation of chemotherapeutics in oncology and antiarrhythmics in cardiology have become extremely comprehensive, resulting in the growing compartmentalization of internal medicine. Patients benefit from these developments and physicians should respect that. The time required for postgraduate training reflects the enormous range of areas—and an issue that is the subject of ongoing debate. Postgraduate training takes three years in the United States and five years plus subsequent subspecialization in European countries. It is safe to say that today no physician is likely to be able to cover the entire spectrum of internal medicine but instead must specialize in certain areas.

In Western countries, internal medicine has split into different areas without the official acceptance of the medical community as a whole. It is nearly impossible for any hospital today to provide care in all specialty areas of internal medicine. Generally, there is an internal medicine department that covers gastroenterology, cardiology, and pulmonology. These areas constitute the traditional polyclinic and can provide care for the majority of patients. The word *polyclinic* is derived from the Greek word *polis,* which means "city." It refers to the traditional city hospital. Other medical historians claim that the word *polyclinic* is derived from the Greek word *polys*, which means "many" or "much." This would apply to a hospital or department that treats many different cases and their origins.

In modern times, most people die of cardiovascular diseases. Some of the most frequent reasons for emergent treatment include myocardial infarction, cardiogenic shock, hypertensive crisis, and metabolic/endocrine causes of coma. Patients may be referred to specialists for treatments or diagnostics, for example, placing a dialysis shunt, specific blood analysis in rheumatic diseases, treatment for thyroid storm, or cancer treatment. Large university hospitals are the exception to this situation. But even here, as we can see in Europe and North America, not all specialty departments exist in one hospital.

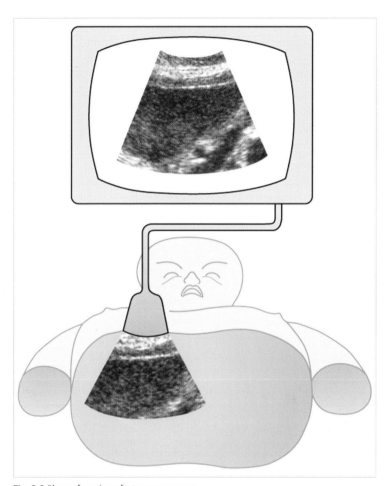

Fig. 3.9 Plane of section of a transverse scan.

Internal medicine has branched into the following areas:
- Cardiology/Angiology/Pulmonology.
- Hematology/Oncology.
- Gastroenterology/Endocrinology.
- Rheumatology.
- Nephrology.
- Emergency medicine/Internal medicine/Intensive care.
- Occupational medicine.

Hospitals maintain different combinations of these areas. For example, many departments may combine nephrology and cardiology or gastroenterology and pulmonology. There is an ongoing discussion about the ideal combination of areas, with no conclusion in sight. What actually matters is that patients receive the optimal level of therapeutic and diagnostic care. The patient should be referred to the proper specialty department when the attending department of internal medicine does not have the necessary capabilities to help them.

While specializing in gastroenterology, pulmonology, or oncology, the physician-to-be learns about diseases specific to these areas along with their highly specialized treatment options. In practice, the physician may not see these types of patients every day because such cases may be directly referred from an outpatient clinic to the specialty center. In my assessment it would be useful to complete the training for general internal medicine at a center for basic and regular care, because these centers usually cover the entire spectrum of internal diseases.

Let's begin with the technical diagnostic methods before moving on to the different sections. In addition to radiographic examinations, which are likely to include thorax imaging as well as CT and MRI, ultrasonography is widely established. Every internist should be able to handle sonographic equipment. In addition, every physician must be capable of interpreting the results obtained via an electrocardiogram (ECG) (**Fig. 3.10**). Every physician must recognize dysrhythmia, ischemia, and infarction.

The diagnostic area of hematology is divided into three sections: morphologic hematology, immunohematology, and hemostaseology. Morphologic hematology involves the microscopic analyses of blood, bone marrow, and smear preparations, as well as biopsies of lymphatic organs. Subtyping of leukemic lymphoma and leukemia is performed via fluorescence-activated cell sorting (FACS). Risk stratification and prognostic assessment are based on cytogenetic methods (genotyping). The main task of immunohematology is human leukocyte antigen (HLA) typing to assess the compatibility assay in organ transplantation. Hemostaseology is focused on the diagnoses of coagulopathies and thrombocytopathies. Therapeutic hematology offers a multilayered spectrum of interventions, including the substitution of coagulation factors, traditional chemotherapy, treatment with biologic agents, and so-called smart drugs that ideally facilitate the specific treatment of malignant hematologic systemic diseases.

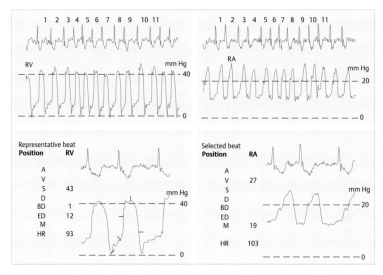

Fig. 3.10 ECG showing hemodynamics in severe tricuspid regurgitation with ventricularization of the right atrial pressure wave.

In the gastroenterology specialty, the student learns about performing gastroscopy, duodenoscopy, endosonographic procedures, colposcopy, and liver biopsy. Pulmonology addresses the use of fiber-optic bronchoscopy, thoracoscopy, and bronchoscopy with and without biopsy sampling. In cardiology, the curriculum includes the use of the following:

- ECGs and evaluating long-term ECGs.
- Echocardiography.
- Ergometry.
- Pacemaker application.
- Coronary intervention via stent implantation.
- Abdominocentesis.
- Sternal puncture.

Regular participation in radiographic demonstrations and pathologic/anatomic conferences, interpretations of laboratory test results, and practicing intensive care, which includes the emergency medicine specialty, are also part of internal medicine training. Particularly in the area of internal medicine—aside from diagnostics and the treatment of internal diseases—technical requirements become ever more important.

3.8.1 Cardiology, Angiology, Pulmonology

Cardiac diseases are differentiated between structural cardiac diseases, such as heart valve defects, coronary heart diseases, and cardiac arrhythmias. Cardiac hypertrophy signifies a mass increase in the size of the heart due to innate cardiac dysfunctions, such as atrial septal defects or ventricular septal defects (**Fig. 3.11**). Pulmonary diseases may also cause cardiac hypertrophy. Hypertrophy leads to dilatation of the heart muscle, an expansion of the heart, with a possible ensuing insufficiency. Students learn during their study of the anatomy of the heart muscle that it constantly depends on an optimal supply of blood and the heart muscle cells require a steady supply of oxygen. Thus, an insufficient supply of blood or oxygen weakens the heart muscle and may result in irreversible damage to heart muscle tissue. Cardiac perfusion via coronary vessels is vital. Coronary vasoconstriction may cause myocardial infarction. In some cases, myocardial infarction may be the result of lifestyle choices (e.g., eating high calorie meals, smoking cigarettes). The origins of coronary insufficiency must be assessed. They may be intracardial, such as a heart valve defect, or extracardial, such as poisoning, anemia, or arteriosclerosis, which is the main type of coronary insufficiency. To assess its origins requires a systemic approach. Partial or complete vascular obstruction can result in myocardial infarction, which signifies the coagulative necrosis of the heart muscle due to an insufficient supply of oxygen. In total, 80% of myocardial infarctions could be avoided by appropriate changes to lifestyle and the recognition of risk factors. In this context, it should be noted that an increasing number of left-heart catheterizations are being performed. Stent implantation has saved many lives; however, due to this, there has been an increase in the number of left-heart catheterizations performed. Ultimately, the point of medicine is the treatment of patients. In the Greater Munich area of Germany, more left-heart catheterizations are performed than in the whole of Great Britain.

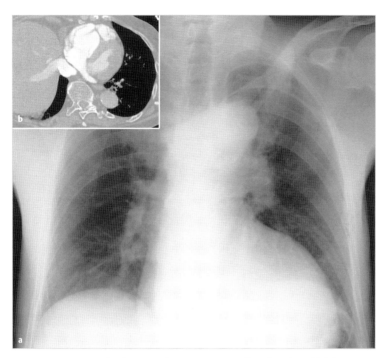

Fig. 3.11 Pressure overload in severe hypertension. Significantly enlarged left heart with pronounced elongation of the aorta along the right cardiac border. There are no signs of decompensation. Deep cardiac waist (**a**). CT demonstrates hypertrophy of the left ventricular wall (**b**). Note the significant congestion in the hepatic veins indicative of left heart failure.

Other large areas of cardiology include: (1) diagnostics and therapy for inflammation, endocarditis caused by bacteria, viruses, or rheumatic fever; and (2) heart valve disorders, such as mitral insufficiency, mitral stenosis, aortic insufficiency, aortic stenosis, tricuspid insufficiency, and pulmonary valve stenosis.

Cardiology also includes therapies for high blood pressure and hypertonia of various origins. Physiology teaches us that pressure receptors in the macula densa of the renal artery help regulate blood pressure. Due to elevated renin secretion, the vasopressor angiotensin is released. Further causes of hypertonia include endocrine hypertonia, for example, as a result of pituitary Cushing's disease, as well as stress and a hectic lifestyle.

In the area of angiology, arteriosclerosis is the central disease picture. Typically, arteriosclerosis is treated via dilatation through the implantation of a stent in the carotid artery or surgical peeling of the arteriosclerotic plaque.

The focus of pulmonology and bronchology includes the various forms of acute and chronic bronchitis, bronchial asthma, various forms of pneumonia, and lung cancer, which has spread rampantly in the Western world. And every year millions of humans die of tuberculosis, which is a leading cause of death around the world (**Fig. 3.12**).

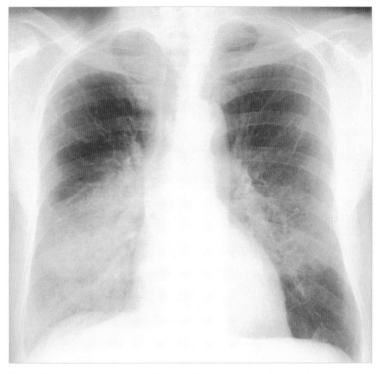

Fig. 3.12 Bronchopneumonia in a 75-year-old man with a long history of chronic obstructive pulmonary disease (COPD). Signs of chronic bronchitis are present with diffuse shadowing and barrel chest with primarily apical emphysema.

3.8.2 Hematology, Oncology

The areas of hematology and oncology include disease diagnostics and treatments for disorders of the blood, blood-building organs, and lymphatic organs. These specialty areas also cover diagnostics and treatment options for hematologic neoplasms, solid tumors, and immunologic and oncologic diseases. In physiology, the student was introduced to blood formation, heme synthesis, and the life-cycle of thrombocytes. Anatomy addressed the makeup of bone marrow. The specific area of hematology includes the classification, diagnosis, and treatment of anemias (e.g., posthemorrhagic anemia, iron deficiency anemia, pernicious anemia, hemolytic anemia, spherocytosis) and elliptocytosis. This specialty also involves autoimmune diseases, such as granulocytopenias, acquired pancytopenias, and granulocytic lesions. There are varying classifications for hemoblastomas. Generally, we make distinctions between undifferentiated, acute, and chronic types of leukemia (**Fig. 3.13**). Genotyping plays an important role in risk stratification. We also differentiate between various types of tumors of the lymph nodes, malignant lymphoma, such as lymphogranulomatosis, Hodgkin's lymphoma, and non-Hodgkin's lymphoma. The specialties of hematology and oncology also include oncologic diagnostics. Professional medical societies have agreed that it should be hematologists that offer cytostatic treatment for all tumors, rather than leaving that responsibility to each individual specialty.

Diagnostics and the treatment of coagulation disorders also belong to the specialty of hematology. This interesting field addresses diseases that many of us know from the historical figures who suffered from them. For example, Queen Victoria of Great Britain had hemophilia, a disorder caused by a genetic defect of the coagulation factor. Due to this heritable condition, many of her male descendants have the disease. Porphyria and porphyrinuria are other types of inherited diseases that were also known to be present in European royal families. It is suggested that Mary Queen of Scots had porphyrinuria, as did her son James and later George III of Great Britain.

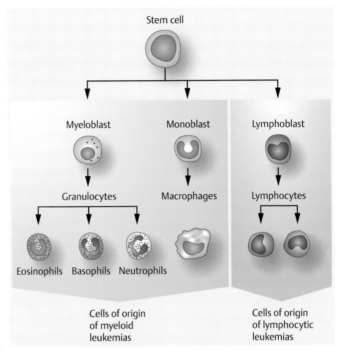

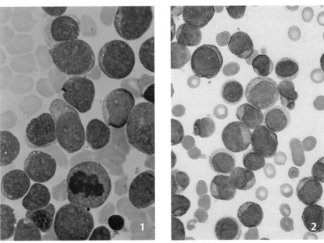

Fig. 3.13 a,b
a Diagram of leukocyte origin: cells of origin for myeloid and lymphocytic leukemias.
b Acute lymphocytic leukemia. Bone marrow: leukemic cells, some containing a nucleolus (1); acute myeloid leukemia. Bone marrow: large polymorphic blasts with multiple nucleoli (2).

3.8.3 Gastroenterology, Endocrinology

Gastroenterology and endocrinology include the treatment of diseases of the esophagus, stomach, intestines, and peritoneum. More specifically, diseases of the esophagus include the formation of a varix following a portal hypertension lesion, acute and chronic esophagitis, and esophageal cancer. In the past few decades, the number of cases of esophageal cancer has considerably increased, although the cause for this rise in incidence is unknown. Stomach disease is another prominent area of gastroenterology, with treatment options for chronic gastritis being a primary challenge for gastroenterologists. Ulcers that require surgery because of gastritis are no longer a common problem—a positive example of therapeutic change! The treatment of a gastric or ventricular ulcers has completely changed as a result of the use of proton pump inhibitors and the discovery of *Helicobacter pylori*. Antibiotics and proton pump inhibitors slow down the production of hydrochloric acid in the stomach lining to a minimum. As a result, the aggressive agent that causes the ulcer is never released. Another focus of stomach diagnostics is gastric cancer, which is decreasing in incidence. Frequently encountered intestinal diseases include inflammatory disorders, such as Crohn's disease and ulcerative colitis, as well as colorectal cancer, which is the third most common type of cancer in US males and females, and the third most common type in males and second most common type in females in Germany. In addition to gastroscopy, colposcopy, and endosonography have become useful diagnostic methods. Capsule endoscopy is of interest, but it is not as common as other methods.

In liver disease, we typically see inflammatory diseases, liver abscesses, and morphologic changes of the liver such as fibrosis or cirrhosis following chronic alcohol use or parasitic infection. In modern times, the causal development of portal hypertension is a complication of liver changes and requires stringent medical supervision. There are primary liver tumors, such as the hepatocellular carcinoma and metastasis, particularly from the colorectal area. Therapeutic approaches for liver tumors are manifold and can include resection, coagulation, embolization, and nanotherapy. These methods are debatable, but none has proven particularly successful over another. In the event of liver failure, an alternative approach is liver transplantation. Performed in specialized institutions, results following liver transplantation may be very positive, giving hope to those patients who are seriously ill.

Other important areas in gastroenterology include pancreatic and gallbladder diseases, such as acute cholecystitis and gallstones. The duodenal papilla can be widened and even gallstones removed via a specialized procedure called endoscopic retrograde cholangiopancreatography (ERCP) (**Fig. 3.14**). The main therapeutic areas in pancreatic diseases include acute and chronic pancreatitis, cystic fibrosis, and pancreatic tumors.

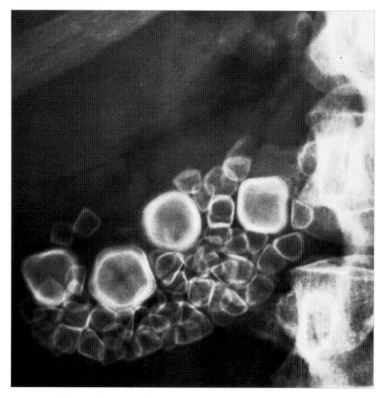

Fig. 3.14 Gallstones shown in radiograph.

In the Western world, one of the most frequently treated diseases seen in internal medicine is type 2 diabetes mellitus. Approximately 400 million people worldwide have some form of diabetes. In addition to controlling the blood sugar level via insulin or insulin analogs, research has shown that the vital glycated hemoglobin value of 6.5% must be maintained in a patient with diabetes. When treating diabetes, it is also important to educate the patient about nutrition, proper body hygiene, and the importance of avoiding foot injuries and ensuing inflammatory diseases to the lower extremities. Intense fluctuations of blood sugar are damaging to all organs but they are particularly detrimental to the kidneys and eyes. This brings me back to my point that some of the most prominent conditions seen in modern medicine are stress and constant "rush." In general, type 2 diabetes is a "lifestyle disease." In the past, humans were mainly the hosts of infectious diseases; today, however, many of us die of diseases of civilization such as type 2 diabetes mellitus, arterial hypertension, and various forms of cancer. Most of these diseases develop slowly and insidiously, which is what makes them so vicious.

Endocrinology comprises diseases of the thyroid gland, such as nodular or multinodular goiter, hyperthyreosis, and Graves' disease. Irish physician Robert James Graves described the triad of symptoms in 1835 (that is, struma, hyperthecosis, and exophthalmos), similarly described in 1840 by Carl Adolph von Basedow. (Graves' disease is known as Basedow's disease in German-speaking countries.) Endocrine conditions also include diseases of the adrenal gland, such as ferrochrome tumors of the adrenal medulla, diseases of the adrenal cortex, and problems with the parathyroid glands. The availability of dialysis has caused a shift in the importance of treatment for hyperparathyroidism. In 1855, the physician Thomas Addison published a text about diseases of the adrenal glands, which he has been connected with ever since (Addison's disease). In fact, many of endocrine diseases are eponymous—that is, they are named after their discoverer. When the majority of these diseases were classified, proper diagnostic techniques were lacking, thus much focus was placed on the description of the findings and then developing an individual conclusion from these findings, which thus led to the logical explanation of the cause of the disease.

3.8.4 Rheumatology

Rheumatology addresses inflammatory and immunologic diseases of the locomotor system and the connective tissue. Thus, rheumatic diseases can be found in every organ in the body. Frequently, the etiologies of such diseases are unknown. Their origins are assumed to be immunologic. Joints are often involved in the disease picture, which places them in the rheumatic spectrum of diseases. The classification of these diseases is still under discussion and subject to change. In the Western world, a uniform classification was agreed upon similar to the classification of diabetes mellitus and psychiatric diseases. Diseases with symptoms of pain or fever, motor disorders involving the joints, eyes, and, in particular, the skin typically have a protracted course. Determining factors can include serologic factors, primarily rheumatoid factors, antibodies against cyclic citrullinated peptides (CCPs), anti-human leukocyte antigens, antinuclear antibodies, and antibodies against cell components. Histocompatibility antigens are currently being discussed as coordinating and prognosis-determining antigens. The most predominant rheumatic diseases include rheumatoid arthritis, systemic lupus erythematous, generalized autoimmune disease with varying tissue damage, scleroderma, vasculitis (e.g., polyarteritis nosoda), Sjögren's syndrome, Still's disease, Reiter's syndrome, rheumatic fever, autoinflammatory syndrome, degenerative arthropathies, and Scheuermann's disease. The application of biologic agents has produced a fundamental change within rheumatic therapies. In recent years, specific chemotherapeutics were developed much like in the field of hemato-oncology. Complementary to cortisone therapy, they improve the course of the disease and quality of life for patients with rheumatic disorders.

3.8.5 Nephrology

Nephrology includes the diagnosis and therapy of kidney diseases, renal hypertension, renal replacement therapy, and dialysis procedures, including peritoneal dialysis. The origins of renal diseases are manifold. In addition to congenital diseases such as cystic kidney and aplasia, significant disorders include various types of glomerulonephritis, pyelonephritis, and interstitial nephritis. Pyelonephritis is the bacterial inflammation of the renal tissue and is frequently caused by bacteria rising from the urinary tract, possibly resulting in abscesses or urosepsis. Classic signs of inflammation include fever, tenderness of the renal bed, and leukocytosis (advanced stage). Those are certain indicators for pyelonephritis. Diagnosis requires clinical examination, ultrasonography, and intravenous pyelogram. The therapy of choice is treatment with a broad-spectrum antibiotic (e.g., cephalosporin, aminoglycoside). Urosepsis is differentiated from pyelonephritis based on a primary outbreak of a urologic infection due to the presence of kidney stones or hematogenous dissemination during which the classic signs of inflammation, such as fever, chills, leukocytosis, tachycardia, and possibly septic shock, will be present. Antibiosis is the gold standard of therapy. Antibiotic susceptibility must be considered.

Urosepsis must be differentiated from tuberculosis of the kidney, which can be a neglected diagnosis in Western Europe. The causative agent is *Mycobacterium tuberculosis*, which is widespread in Eastern Europe. Immediate treatment is essential due to the destruction of kidney tissue caused by the spread of *M. tuberculosis*—called caseous cell necrosis. Traditional antituberculotic drugs include isoniazid, rifampicin, streptomycin, and ethambutol. Tuberculosis of the kidney must be differentiated from abacterial interstitial nephritis, which is caused by the use of drugs such as cytostatics, nonsteroidal antirheumatics, and other toxic substances. Therapy involves avoiding the primary causes of the disease.

Renal cell carcinoma (also called adenocarcinoma of the kidney or hypernephroma) and Wilms' tumor (also called nephroblastoma) are types of kidney cancer typically found in the pediatric population. Similar to the other oncologic areas, the tumor–node–metastasis (TNM) classification applies. Crucial to successful and efficient treatment are early diagnosis and tumor removal. Nephrology includes the proper indication for likely candidates for kidney transplantation in cases of kidney failure, metabolic disorders with stone formation, and nodular glomerulosclerosis, also known as Kimmelstiel–Wilson syndrome, caused by type 2 diabetes mellitus (**Fig. 3.15**).

Most disorders of the kidney lead to chronic kidney insufficiency and the imbalances of various metabolic processes. Therefore, nephrologists are experts in the field of metabolism. Adequate hormone and mineral replacement therapy—depending on the kidneys—may prevent secondary complications and possibly delay the need for dialysis.

3.8.6 Emergency Medicine and Intensive Care

Emergency medicine is taking on greater significance, particularly in internal medicine. Cardiopulmonary resuscitation as part of basic life support (BLS) should be part of the armamentarium of every health care professional. Emergency care includes treatment of angina pectoris, hypertensive crisis, myocardial infarction, and respiratory emergencies, such as bronchial asthma and pneumothorax, among other conditions.

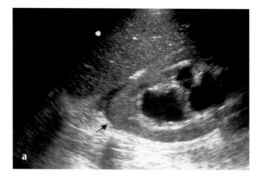

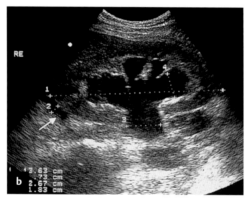

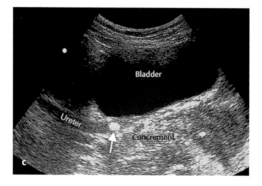

Fig. 3.15 (a–c) Sonographic findings in a patient with acute right-sided renal colic.
a, b Evidence of acute urinary tract obstruction on the right side with rupture of the fornix (arrows).
c The cause is a concrement of approximately 8 × 5 mm located prevesically, approximately 5–8 mm in front of the ostium (arrow).

Diabetic coma is one of the most frequently seen endocrine emergencies. Emergencies due to intoxication also loom large. The numbers of lead, arsenic, or mercury poisonings are decreasing, but the number of drug-induced emergencies is rapidly growing. During their studies of internal medicine, students must learn to recognize hallucinogens and intoxications due to opiates, amphetamines, sedatives, cocaine, and cannabis. In the United States, emergency medicine is its own specialty area; however, in Western Europe, it is generally considered a subspecialty. For example, in Germany it is covered by the optional postgraduate internal medicine training. In North America, geographic structures may not allow every small community to have its own emergency center. In rural areas, helicopters may be the fastest method of transportation available. For this reason, emergency departments have been established in which patients receive immediate treatment. Following initial treatment in the emergency department, patients are then typically referred to specialists as necessary. This system has been well developed and refined in the United States, and European countries have begun to adopt it. Blanket coverage of emergency care exists in Western Europe via emergency ambulances and helicopters. In addition, European hospitals are equipped with emergency wards to separate emergent and nonemergent patients; doing so gives health care professionals the advantage that less severe diseases or injuries can be adequately treated and, concurrently, emergency physicians can refer patients with serious diseases directly to their colleagues from other specialties.

3.8.7 Occupational Medicine

Occupational medicine can be considered the interface between medicine and the working environment. The specific conditions of a person in his or her working environment are analyzed by an occupational medicine specialist, who then helps to work with the patient to minimize potential risks or dangers. Typical examples include wearing a protective helmet on construction sites, wearing white coats in chemical laboratories, and wearing eye protection, face protection, or both during benchwork.

Occupational medicine focuses on the activities of people working with hazardous materials, such as toxic substances in laboratories, and on the large group of traditional occupational diseases. The long list of these ailments includes the following:

- Allergies (first introduced in the pathology and dermatology units).
- Hand eczema (commonly seen, e.g., in hairdressers and painters).

- Lead poisoning in people in contact with gasoline or those in the petroleum industry.
- Chrome, cadmium, or manganese poisoning and their prevention.
- Diseases caused by carcinogenic substances, such as asbestos, which may trigger pleural mesothelioma.
- Carcinoma caused by polycyclic hydrocarbons used in various industrial processes.

Occupational medicine also includes the protection of noise pollution or ionizing radiation at the work site and the provision of adequate light in the work place. This requires the collaboration of radiotherapists and radiation physicists. In hospitals, specially trained personnel alone are permitted to work in the departments of diagnostic radiology, radiotherapy, and nuclear medicine. Twice a year they must undergo occupational health examinations. Furthermore, at least twice a year they wear dosimeters on their coats to measure radiation exposure. Occupational medicine is far removed from direct curative medicine and patient contact. However, there is a particular appeal to the collaboration of medicine and the working world.

3.9 Pediatrics

Pediatrics includes the prevention, diagnosis, and therapy of all physical and psychological diseases, behavioral syndromes, and developmental disorders of infants, toddlers, and children up to the completion of their somatic development (**Fig. 3.16**). In recent years, the field of pediatrics has been rapidly developing in the areas of oncology and neonatology. There is a need for highly specialized pediatricians in both of these subspecialties. Extensive knowledge and experience are both necessary to provide optimal care to the pediatric population. In the Western world, large children's hospitals with 100 beds or more in which children were treated for tuberculosis or diphtheria belong to the past. As time goes by, children's hospitals are closing because many diseases can now be treated in outpatient clinics and systematic vaccinations have reduced the outbreak of many diseases as compared with 50 years ago.

Pediatric diseases and their range of treatment options have undergone considerable changes, specifically in the area of childhood hemato-oncology. In this field, pediatric oncologists exclusively focus on tumoral

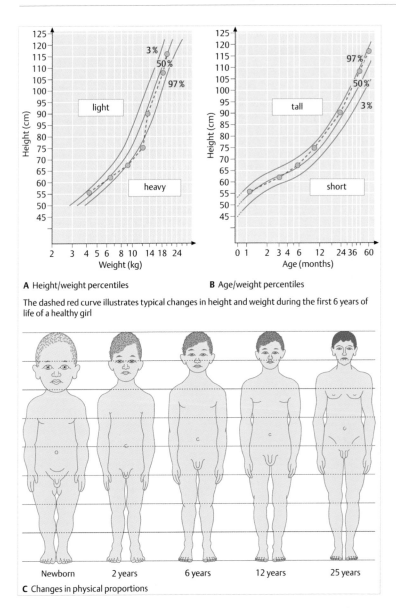

A Height/weight percentiles

B Age/weight percentiles

The dashed red curve illustrates typical changes in height and weight during the first 6 years of life of a healthy girl

Newborn   2 years   6 years   12 years   25 years

C Changes in physical proportions

Fig. 3.16 Chart of the various child development stages. The neonatal period is followed by infancy, followed by early childhood, late childhood/preadolescence, and adolescence.

diseases of the blood, the hematopoietic organs, and the lymphatic system. Chemotherapy, interdisciplinary collaboration, and bone marrow transplantations are emphasized in this pediatric area and include the following:

- Tumor therapy and the coordinated efforts of radiotherapists, pathologists, pediatric surgeons, and pediatrics—similar to the therapy for adulthood tumors.
- Dependable indications for bone marrow transplantations due to the sensitivity of the bone marrow.
- Follow-up and rehabilitation care after tumor diseases occurring in childhood.

A second area of emphasis is neonatology. In Western countries, it has become common practice for gynecologists to monitor the birthing process; the newborn child is then immediately passed on to a pediatric or neonatologist if medical care is required. The involvement of the neonatologist revolves around the following activities:

- Regular examination of cardiovascular and respiratory functions.
- Checking the acid–base and water equilibrium of the newborn.
- Checking temperature regulation.
- If necessary, volume therapy and enteral and parenteral nutrition.
- Treatment of life-threatening infections of the newborn with highly pathogenic agents.
- Medical care for premature infants with a birth weight below 2 kg.

In the past, the field of pediatrics had made enormous progress in the area of viral infections and the general treatment of gastroenterological diseases in childhood. Violent offenses against children are on the rise in the Western world due to demographic developments. For this reason, violence and addiction prevention programs are essential subjects of pediatric training. It is important to recognize and prevent violence against children. Doing so requires the ability to provide sexual counseling and be able to sensibly work with public authorities in the event of suspected child abuse.

The third area of emphasis is pediatric cardiology, which is an area focused on drug treatment and follow-up of congenital and acquired cardiac diseases. Childhood cardiac arrhythmias, as well as vital echocardiographic and Doppler examinations and necessary ECG, are part of everyday life for pediatricians.

The fourth newly developed area of emphasis within pediatrics is neuropediatrics, which focuses on the treatment of tumors in the central and peripheral nervous system, motor disorders, and post-traumatic or inflammatory changes in the central nervous system.

Typically, the field of pediatrics is subdivided within large pediatric institutions. General pediatric wards in large hospitals or in rural areas usually cover the treatment of infectious and gastroenterological conditions. In general, behavioral problems in children are increasing steadily, especially in urban environments with a lack of stable family structure. Children can be affected by environmental conditions, stress, and family problems, thus, child and adolescent psychiatry is yet another area crucial to pediatrics.

As we can see, pediatrics is a most relevant and interesting field that can give the practitioner a deeply satisfying purpose. However, modern pediatricians working in a pediatric clinic in the Western world should not conduct every pediatric therapy possible. Young patients are more likely to benefit when pediatricians focus on their specialty areas and approaches described above.

In pediatrics we encounter some peculiarities due to the ages of these patients. The clinical interview and patient history is as important in pediatrics as in other areas, but, depending on how young the patient is, the interview and history may be via a third party. Frequently, there are two "patients," the child and the parent(s). Particularly in pediatrics, it is important to be professionally competent and approach patients in the most appropriate way. For example, a urologist and a surgeon are likely to approach the same patient in very different ways. However, when helping to care for young patients, it is important to exercise caution and not intimidate them. Therapeutic success depends to a considerable degree on verbal and nonverbal language, diction, tone, and the pediatrician's appearance. When taking a child's medical history, it is essential to take the family history into consideration. The medical history of a toddler's development provides important clues to whether the child is appropriately thriving. The student should watch for specific signs, such as acoustic and visual attention after 4 to 6 weeks, sitting without help after 6 to 8 months, unassisted walking after 12 to 18 months, speaking single words by the end of the first year, and controlling bowel functions after 18 months, among other growth milestones. The medical history of reflexes, such as the grasping, Moro, or glabellar tap reflex, offer indications for possible neurologic disorders. Medical history taking and performing a clinical examination are both vital in young patients. Examination of a newborn centers on the stability of the hip joints, skin color, blood flow to the extremities, head circumference, and the exclusion of prenatal infections.

Modern pediatrics includes being knowledgeable about genetics and congenital diseases such as autosomal chromosome aberration, Turner's syndrome, Klinefelter's syndrome, and others. Pediatric diseases also include metabolic diseases such as histidinuria and urea cycle disorder. There is also a broad spectrum of gastrointestinal diseases. The rather common pedicle torsion and axial rotation of the intestines may cause volvulus, a total constriction of the intestines that completely halts the blood supply. These disorders usually begin without preceding symptoms other than the innocuous stomachache, yet some cases are fatal. It takes professional experience to differentiate harmless stomach pain from a life-threatening condition.

The most frequent childhood bacterial infection is acute otitis media, and bronchial asthma is the most frequent childhood pulmonary disease. This applies particularly to Western urban areas and numbers are increasing. The frequent disposition for pulmonary diseases is thought to be due to environmental pollution caused by carbon dioxide emissions. Moreover, many children do not spend enough time outdoors or exercising. In the West, societal and lifestyle changes have led to blatant maldevelopment. Bronchial asthma, being overweight, type 2 diabetes mellitus, and psychosomatic irregularities are only some of the diseases within the scope of pediatrics that pose challenges to today's and future pediatricians.

In the infectious diseases specialty, meningococcal meningitis, diphtheria, tetanus, and pertussis rank at the top. Increased numbers of immigrants have produced a resurgence of some of these old diseases. For example, an increasing number of foreign-born people from Latin America and Asia have been exposed to tuberculosis and represent nearly 47% of US cases of tuberculosis, a disease that had been under control since the 1950s (American Lung Association 2010).

Pediatric surgery is also a subspecialty of pediatrics and includes anorectal malformations, hypoplasias, intestinal diseases, abdominal tumors, and hernias. Medical students wishing to belong to this field of study must specialize early on in their careers. Those who are fascinated by surgery and eager to help young patients will find fulfillment in this subspeciality.

3.10 Dermatology

Dermatology is characterized by the visual recognition of disease more than any other field of medicine. The dermatologist must be trained to perceive even the minutest of changes of the skin.

The primary purpose of the skin is to protect the body. The entire skin surface of an adult covers approximately 2 m². Dermatology also includes the treatment of mucous membranes, subcutaneous tissue, and skin appendages, such as the hair and nails. Knowledge of the skin structure is crucial to understanding the pathophysiologic origins of skin diseases. The skin is divided into the epidermis, which is the outer layer with several keratinizing squamous epithelia, the dermis, and the subcutis (**Fig. 3.17**). The anatomy of the skin can be learned relatively easily, but it is critical in dermatology to master differential diagnoses and exact descriptions of visual findings and to carefully approach the final diagnosis. Dermatologic diagnostics and therapy include the visual examination and palpation of the diseased skin, as well as pathology, modern laboratory diagnostic tools, and serology. In particular, dermatology requires the thorough description of visual findings, which is an integrative factor of diagnosis, and must follow strict criteria. The skin is more than a protective organ against radiation and heat. It also functions as an acidic coat that protects the body with a pH value between 4 and 6 and regulates the water balance. Furthermore, due to the skin's sensitivity to touch and temperature, it has communicative qualities. The skin regulates body temperature and is where vitamin D is synthesized. In viral diseases, for example through the human herpesvirus, we can usually see unilateral changes of the back or abdominal skin along the path of a nerve. We can recognize diseases of the skin or the tissues below according to the change in color of the skin. Red indicates hemorrhaging, black suggests necrosis, and yellow can point toward purulence. The skin provides many indications, such as pressure pain and itching (constant or intermittent, only on certain days or upon contact with certain objects, plants, or animals). All these indications are important, especially when diagnosing allergies.

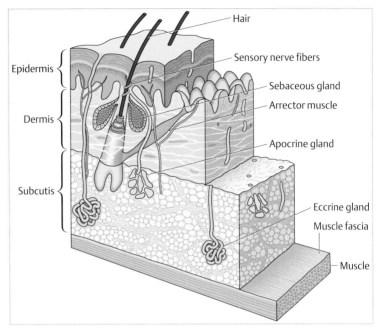

Fig. 3.17 Three-dimensional diagram of the skin.

At the beginning of a dermatologic consultation, the general condition of the skin is examined. Is it dry, greasy, wrinkled, dull, or shiny? Skin changes, also called efflorescences, can be singular, multiple, extensive, stripe-like, segmentally confluent across the entire body, or herpetiform. These characteristic descriptions are crucial to diagnoses. Specifically in cases of skin efflorescences, and all other skin diseases in general, both the patient and his or her family histories must be considered. We generally differentiate between primary efflorescences, such as spots, papules, nodules, follicles, blisters, or pustules. Blisters can turn into scabs, which would be considered a secondary efflorescence. Pustules can turn into blisters or scars and circulatory disorders into ulcers. The strict classification and differentiation between primary and secondary efflorescences facilitates the accurate diagnosis of the dermatologic disease. For example, the physician may be presented with a patient whose skin has changed to the color white, and this change has segmentally spread across the entire body. This patient's history must be taken because it can help lead to a diagnosis. A patient who spends a lot of time outdoors (and thus has increased sun exposure) may develop hyperkeratosis, which is increased cornification. Many older adults may have cyanosis of the lips. Blue discoloration of the skin can also be seen in patients with cardiac disorders; in such cases, the blood lacks oxygen. Sometimes the sclerae are affected. Physicians may encounter white skin and white mucous membranes in all types of anemias, as well as vitiligo. In addition to red or blue skin discoloration, we may see yellow discoloration in icteric disorders, which are liver or gallbladder diseases. It may be helpful to place patients in front of a blue background; doing so will help the physician detect even the slightest yellowish discoloration.

Hair and nails are also part of the dermatologic examination. They too can give indications about nutritional disorders, poor hygiene, hormonal disorders, fungal growth, or systemic diseases.

Sexually transmitted infections, which were known in the past as venereal diseases, also belong to the field of dermatology. We have already learned about allergology in pathology and biochemistry, but it is also a dermatologic subspecialty. Surgical therapy is another—specifically tumor surgery. Dermatologic tumor surgery involves the removal of cancers such as basal cell carcinoma, squamous cell carcinoma, melanoma, and sentinel lymph nodes. In the event of venous insufficiency, a surgical intervention called stripping—also part of dermatology—may be necessary.

In recent years, the number of cosmetic surgeries has risen considerably. These types of surgeries include scar revision and liposuction. These surgical interventions must be accompanied by a detailed consultation with a surgical dermatologist or a similar professional.

As we can see, a multitude of dermatologic diseases and pathophysiologic causative agents exist for various forms of disease. In the field of dermatology, frequently there is a tedious, step-by-step path to reach the correct diagnosis. Adequate therapy depends on the exact diagnosis of the skin disease and on the physician's understanding of pathophysiology. This is the case in nearly all medical areas, but it is most crucial in dermatology.

Sun bathing—spending extended periods of time in sunny places, and "working on a tan" via natural or unnatural light—are all behaviors likely to have led to the rise in incidence of malignant melanoma. The responsibilities of the dermatologist are not limited to exacting the correct diagnoses of chronic atopic diseases alone, such as psoriasis or viral, bacterial, or mycotic diseases, but also include preventive measures. In most cases, dermatologists should explain to patients why sunscreen is necessary and recommend a cancer check-up through dermatoscopy.

Physicians must be capable of recognizing chronic cuticle disorders, such as cornification disorders, and all types of eczema. Every physician should also be able to diagnose malignant diseases of the pigment system, which include malignant melanomas, and refer patients to dermatologic specialistsif they require additional care.

3.11 Neurology

Just as in every other medical field, the neurologic examination and history represent the foundation of the physician's ability to make the correct diagnosis. However, in the field of neurology, diagnosing is a demanding intellectual challenge and patient outcomes depend on a thorough medical history, specific findings on clinical examination, and, to perhaps an even higher degree, on the experience of the neurologist. We differentiate between neurologic symptoms, which are deviations from physiologic processes, and neurologic syndromes, which represent the combination of different symptoms. This is considered a neurologic deviation from the normal.

Part of the neurologic examination is the physical examination of the patient, which includes reviewing his or her state of consciousness, cranial nerves, motor functions, extrapyramidal motor function, sensitivity, reflexes, cerebellar signs, as well as an orienting neuropsychological examination and a general psychiatric exploration. The neurologist is frequently the first person to diagnosis psychiatric changes and will then refer the patient to the psychiatrist. Standard neurologic diagnostics include symptoms of intracranial pressure, various coma stages, and symptoms of paraplegia, such as spinal shock as one of the five shock conditions, complete paraplegia, or symptoms of spinal artery shock in the setting of aortic aneurism.

Laboratory tests, such as a complete blood count and liquor (cerebrospinal fluid) diagnostics, are of great importance in this field. Evoked potentials, measurements of nerve conduction velocity, electromyography, and findings on muscle biopsy are also part of neurologic diagnostics. Neurologic imaging procedures include conventional X-ray imaging, particularly of the spine in cases of changes in intervertebral disks, CT, MRI, angiography, PET, and transcranial Doppler ultrasonography, which is an established approach in cases of cerebral circulatory disorders (**Fig. 3.18**). Neurology also involves the diagnosis and therapy of neurologic diseases, whereas neurosurgery is concerned with surgical intervention in peripheral or central nervous system diseases (e.g., surgeries for cerebral tumors, cerebral hemorrhaging, intervertebral disk disorders). Stereotactic intervention can serve diagnostic purposes or it may be performed to implant devices in the brain (e.g., for people with Parkinson's disease or another motor disorder). This type of intervention is an interdisciplinary approach between neurology and neurosurgery. The most frequently performed surgeries in small children include shunt implants in the event of hydrocephalus, which is the pathologic expansion of the subarachnoid space in the central nervous system, or surgical correction in the event of spina bifida.

Another wide range of neurologic diagnostics includes inflammatory changes of the nervous system following viral infection—particularly encephalitis caused by the human herpesvirus but rarely following measles—bacterial infections, or immunologic diseases of the nervous system such as multiple sclerosis. Beyond diagnostics, antibiotic therapy, or therapy with cortisone, immunoglobulins, or immunotherapeutics (e.g., multiple sclerosis), are common modern standards. Traumatic brain injury belongs to the specialties of neurology and neurosurgery. Particularly in the event of motor vehicle collisions or falls from great heights, both therapy and rehabilitation are included in treatment plans.

Neurology is a field with great potential for growth because of the ever-increasing life expectancy of people living in the Western hemisphere. Chronic diseases, such as cerebral circulatory disorders, along with stroke, neurodegenerative diseases, including Alzheimer's and Parkinson's diseases, will continue to grow in incidence. Combine unhealthy lifestyle choices with these conditions and the medical student will begin to understand why the medical community is seeing more and more patients present with circulatory disorders and neurologic manifestations. Here again, neurology and neurosurgery work hand in hand. An artificial extraintracranial arterial anastomosis allows partial compensation of circulatory disorders.

Apart from degenerative brain diseases (e.g., Huntington's disease), Parkinson's disease is the domain of neurologic diagnostics and therapy. In addition to drug therapy, physical therapy is an important part of the treatment of Parkinson's disease. Many highly specialized institutions exist that can offer individual therapies for patients with this neurologic disease. It is also worth noting that many people with Parkinson's disease are elderly; therefore, multidisciplinary collaboration is required—and is a leading example for many of the therapeutic approaches used in medicine.

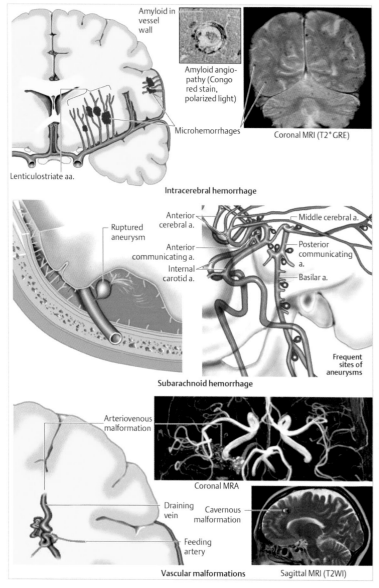

Fig. 3.18 Intracerebral hemorrhage, subarachnoid hemorrhage, vascular malformations.

The varying types of epilepsy make up yet another specialty of neurology. We differentiate between primary generalized seizures, including grand mal and petit mal seizures, and focal seizures, including simple-

and complex-focal seizures, which can also result in grand mal seizures. Gaius Julius Caesar and Vincent van Gogh are two famous people who were thought to have had epilepsy.

The Writings of Famous Figures from Medicine

Harvey Williams Cushing specialized in neurosurgery and postulated that brain surgery required highly specialized technology to succeed. He wrote two wonderful diaries (Cushing 1936, 1944) and there are several biographies about his life, for example, Thomson (1950) and Bliss (2005). South African Christiaan Barnard, the famous heart surgeon who performed the world's first successful heart transplantation, wrote an autobiography well worth reading (Barnard 1969). The biographies of Rudolf Virchow, a pathologist, and Ferdinand Sauerbruch, a surgeon, are each deeply touching (Schipperges 1994, Goschler 2009, Vasold 1990, Andree 2002, Sauerbruch 1995). Whoever believes that they are the only one having trouble while studying medicine is seriously mistaken. Great physicians have shared this suffering. It is helpful and comforting to read their biographies. It teaches the medical student about history and the development of personality, helping to facilitate some insight into what is really important about being a doctor: love for the work, love and respect for the patient and his or her disease, and the absolute determination to help. I also recommend reading the writings of Lord Moran (Baron Charles McMoran Wilson (1966)), who was Winston Churchill's personal physician. I strongly recommend reading the work of Swiss thanatologist Elisabeth Kuebler-Ross, whose research about the last stages of life, conducted in New York after World War II, was groundbreaking and is now standard reading for every physician. For years she recorded her conversations with the dying. As a result, she described the five stages of dying (denial, anger, bargaining, depression, acceptance) in her famous work, *On Death and Dying* (Kuebler-Ross 1954):

- The first stage involves denial, isolation and shock.
- The second stage follows with "Why me?", anger, and aggression.
- In the third phase the dying person tries to bargain.
- During the fourth phase the patient realizes that he or she will have to part from this life; depression and fear for the partner sets in.
- In the fifth stage the patient accepts his or her fate.

Another domain of neurologists (along with bioethicists) gaining importance is the diagnostics of brain death. Being able to diagnose brain death prior to ischemic injury, for example, is essential to the "dead-donor rule," which posits that vital organs be taken only from an organ donor who is dead but that the operation to remove those organs cannot be the *cause* of such death. Usually, two physicians who work independently from the transplant team must perform this procedure.

As we have learned in physiology, a close interaction of nerves and muscles exists at the motor end plate, which is reflected in modern neurologic diagnostics and therapy. Dystrophic myopathies and inflammatory myopathies are also subjects of neurology.

Daily practice proves that findings on clinical examination can deliver decisive diagnostic arguments. Aside from laboratory results, extensive, well-performed clinical examinations account for more than 60% of a typical diagnosis. One renowned neurosurgeon used to say about patients with severe disk prolapse that "I do not operate on X-rays but on people."

Medical students looking for a challenging nonsurgical subject, who appreciate thoroughness, precise anamneses, and the topical allocation of syndromes, will find the field of neurology to be a great choice of specialty.

3.12 Psychiatry, Psychosomatics, and Psychotherapy

It is always a challenge to write a chapter on psychiatry. Should we begin with Sigmund Freud or Alfred Adler? Or should we go back in history and work our way forward to the latest developments of psychiatry? I prefer the approach of beginning with the subject's position within the entire field of medicine. The German-American medical historian Erwin Ackerknecht put it this way: "One could go as far as to say that there is not a single case of illness to which a psychiatrist could not contribute" (Ackerknecht 1967). Or, as the Austrian psychosomatic specialist Wolfgang Wesiack, puts it: "There are psychological and somatic findings in every patient. From this vantage point, every patient is psychosomatically ill, whether he suffers from a plain neurosis or a primarily organic disease" (Wesiack 1988). To me, this is a good introduction to psychiatry because it expresses the significance and value of psychiatry within the framework of modern medicine. In general, every physician should have a basic understanding of psychiatry. Psychiatry differs considerably from subjects such as surgery or ophthalmology; moreover, the courses of disease can make it a relatively difficult subject to study. Psychiatry is highly differentiated and complex. As far as symptomology is concerned, the medical student will encounter differing developments, opinions, and professional stances during their study of the field.

This leads us to the foundations of psychiatry and psychotherapy. In the past, eponyms were used to name schizophrenic diseases (e.g., schizophrenia was a term coined by Swiss psychiatrist Paul Eugen Bleuler and was originally termed "Bleuler's disease"). There are two modern-day classifications of psychiatric diseases: the *Diagnostic and Statistical Manual of Mental Disorders, Fifth Edition (DSM-5)*, which is published by the American Psychiatric Association, and the *International Statistical Classification of Diseases and Related Health Problems* (ICD-10) by the World Health Organization, according to which there are 11 groups of psychiatric diseases or disorders, for example organic disorders, schizophrenia, and behavioral disorders in children and in adolescents. This classification is generally accepted and applied in practice in many Western countries. Pathology is the only other medical field in which classification of diseases has developed to that extent.

Along with disease classification and the psychiatric consultation (patient history, clinical examination), clinical psychopathological findings are the psychiatrist's most important tools. Additional significant diagnostic tools include laboratory tests, electroencephalogram (EEG), brain mapping, validated psychological test procedures, and select imaging methods (radiography, CT, MRI, and PET [used mainly in cases of degenerative cerebral diseases]). Psychological test procedures are used for diagnostic purposes in children and adolescents. The Wechsler Intelligence Scale for Children (WISC) is an example of this approach. It is essential to recognize and classify certain symptoms and syndromes in order to diagnose and treat psychiatric diseases. Psychiatrists describe psychopathological findings such as dynamics and drive, as in stuporous change in motor function in which the patient remains blank and rigid; nervousness with unintended, involuntary, and uncontrollable movements; changes in speech, such as paralogy, in which sentence structure and thought coordination do not follow logic; abnormal memory disorders of deficits; and self-identity disorders, such as derealization and depersonalization.

Psychiatric emergencies are typically cases of acute psychotic conditions in which a person has lost his or her sense of reality. People with these conditions are generally treated with neuroleptics and benzodiazepine derivatives to control these psychiatric crises and to help prevent possible suicide attempts.

Treatment approaches to psychiatric diseases may include directive procedures, psychodynamic psychotherapy, cognitive behavioral therapy, or family therapy, as well as various pharmacologic therapeutic options. We were introduced to antidepressants in pharmacology. Sometimes they may be appropriate for patients with obsessive-compulsive disorder, anxiety disorders, or personality disorders. In some cases, neuroleptics and tranquilizers may also be useful (e.g., neuroleptics for schizophrenic psychoses, schizoaffective psychoses, acute states of agitation, delusions, and bipolar disorders; tranquilizers for dissipating anxiety and stress). The knowledge of drug–drug interactions is crucial, as is the limited indications among patients who are pregnant and the therapeutic range and adverse events of psychiatric medications.

Psychiatrists may be given the vital task of recognizing and treating suicidal tendencies in their patients; thus, they must learn to interpret their patient's words, actions, and gestures and integrate them into a holistic picture of their patient. Just as surgeons must be trained to recognize different tissues so they know what type of suture to choose for a particular tendon or vein, psychiatrists must learn to recognize the alarm signals for suicidal tendencies. The Austrian psychiatrist Erwin Ringel (1983) described a presuicidal syndrome consisting of confinement, inhibited self-aggression, and suicidal fantasies (which may ultimately be carried out). More than one-third of patients who commit suicide have attempted suicide several times before. In many countries, United States and Germany among them, more people die committing suicide than in traffic accidents every year.

In Western countries, various substances are common causes of addiction. Worldwide, alcohol is the leading cause of addictive behavior (**Fig. 3.19**). Social pressures or insidious habit are frequently the cause of addictive behaviors. For example, people who smoke are more likely to have family members who smoke than those who do not smoke. Environment is yet another determining factor in addictions. Stress, hectic days, and the pressure to succeed at the workplace may prompt addictive behavior. People who cannot calm down in the evening may find a glass of wine very helpful (because alcohol is a depressant); however, with time one glass may turn into two, or three, thus potentially leading to addiction. American physiologist Elvin Morton Jellinek (1960) summarized the stages toward alcohol addiction in four steps:

1. Prealcoholic stage, with drinking for relief.
2. Prodromal stage, with increased tolerance and memory lapses.

3. The critical stage, with compulsive drinking and loss of control.
4. Chronic stage, with lowered tolerance, physical, emotional, and social decline, psychosis, and delirium.

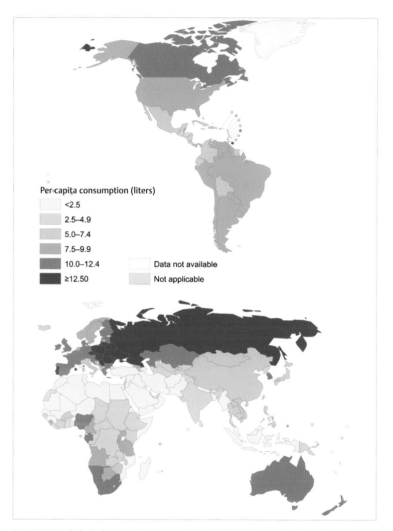

Fig. 3.19 Total alcohol per capita consumption (2010) (15+ years; in liters of pure alcohol).[1]

---

1 Reproduced, with the permission of the publisher, from WHO. Global Status Report on Alcohol and Health 2014. Fig. 2. Geneva: World Health Organization; 2014:29. Available at: http://www.who.int/substance_abuse/publications/global_alcohol_report/en. Accessed November 10, 2014.

The regular consumption of alcohol with the initially accompanying feeling of euphoria may lead to considerable somatic consequences, including the development of acute or chronic pancreatitis, gastritis, reflux esophagitis, fatty liver disease, liver cirrhosis with esophageal varices, and frequent skin infections due to poor hygiene. Long-term alcohol consumption may result in chronic conditions such as degenerative cerebral diseases, including Korsakoff's syndrome (a memory disorder with confabulation tendencies) and the acute form of Wernicke's encephalopathy in combination with vitamin B1 deficiency due to poor nutrition. The latter is characterized by psycho-organic syndrome with disorientation, unsteady gait or standing (cerebellar ataxia), eye movement disorders, and ophthalmoplegia. Psychological secondary diseases include acute delirium, epilepsy, abnormal reactions with complete disinhibition, and pathologic intoxication, which is an epileptic fugue state caused by alcohol. Therapy in these cases starts with immediate and complete sobriety. This form of withdrawal takes place in a clinic with an internal medicine department and intensive care and may be followed by therapy at an outpatient rehabilitation center and psychotherapy at an addiction counseling facility.

People often become addicted to prescription medications. People who are older may become addicted to benzodiazepines and other similar sleeping pills such as zopiclone. Others may become addicted to illicit drugs, as well as nicotine, or opioids such as tramadol. While the number of tobacco consumers decreases, the number of (illegal) drug users increases, especially in Western urban areas (United Nations Office on Drugs and Crime 2014). Abusive consumption can include cannabis, amphetamines, cocaine, phencyclidine, methamphetamine, and illicit hallucinogens (**Table 3.1**, **Table 3.2**). Therapy may consist of inpatient withdrawal, inpatient rehabilitation, and long-term outpatient psychotherapeutic care.

Table 3.1 Annual prevalence of the use of cannabis, opioids and opiates, by region[2]

Region or subregion	Cannabis					
	Number (thousands)			Prevalence (percentage)		
	Best Estimate	Lower	Upper	Best Estimate	Lower	Upper
Africa	44,560	19,860	57,530	7.5	3.3	9.7
East Africa	6,210	2,070	10,580	4.1	1.4	7.1
North Africa	5,610	2,850	8,670	4.3	2.2	6.6
Southern Africa	4,230	2,950	7,700	5.0	3.5	9.1
West and Central Africa	28,510	11,990	30,570	12.4	5.2	13.3
Americas	51,820	51,090	53,300	8.1	8.0	8.4
Caribbean	690	320	1,810	2.5	1.2	6.6
Central America	680	660	720	2.6	2.5	2.7
North America	35,230	35,040	35,430	11.2	11.2	11.3
South America	15,220	15,080	15,340	5.7	5.6	5.7
Asia	54,610	28,900	88,100	1.9	1.0	3.1
Central Asia and Transcaucasia	1,870	1,310	2,200	3.5	2.4	4.1
East and South-East Asia	10,140	5,910	23,440	0.6	0.4	1.5
Near and Middle East/ South West Asia	9,390	5,450	13,200	3.4	2.0	4.8
South Asia	33,210	16,230	49,240	3.5	1.7	5.2
Europe	24,000	23,220	24,800	4.3	4.2	4.5
Eastern and South-Eastern Europe	5,470	4,750	6,210	2.4	2.1	2.7
Western and Central Europe	18,530	18,460	18,590	5.7	5.7	5.7
Oceania	2,650	2,220	3,540	10.8	9.1	14.5
Global Estimate	**177,600**	**125,300**	**227,300**	**3.8**	**2.7**	**4.9**

Continued ▶

2 United Nations Office on Drugs and Crime. World Drug Report 2014 (United Nations Publication, Sales No. E.14.XI.7), Annex I, S. X. © United Nations, June 2014. Available at: http://www.unodc.org/wdr2014. Accessed September 23, 2014.

Table 3.1 (Continued)

| Region or subregion | Opioids | | | | | |
| | Number (thousands) | | | Prevalence (percentage) | | |
	Best Estimate	Lower	Upper	Best Estimate	Lower	Upper
Africa	1,930	900	3,140	0.3	0.2	0.5
East Africa	250	90	1,100	0.2	0.1	0.7
North Africa	320	130	520	0.2	0.1	0.4
Southern Africa	340	230	360	0.4	0.3	0.4
West and Central Africa	1,020	440	1,150	0.4	0.2	0.5
Americas	14,440	14,210	14,710	2.3	2.2	2.3
Caribbean	100	60	190	0.4	0.2	0.7
Central America	40	40	50	0.2	0.1	0.2
North America	13,460	13,320	13,600	4.3	4.2	4.3
South America	830	800	870	0.3	0.3	0.3
Asia	11,920	9,040	15,380	0.4	0.3	0.5
Central Asia and Transcaucasia	470	460	490	0.9	0.9	0.9
East and South-East Asia	3,370	2,530	4,740	0.2	0.2	0.3
Near and Middle East/ South West Asia	5,190	3,880	6,540	1.9	1.4	2.4
South Asia	2,890	2,170	3,610	0.3	0.2	0.4
Europe	4,010	3,930	4,100	0.7	0.7	0.7
Eastern and South-Eastern Europe	2,800	2,790	2,810	1.2	1.2	1.2
Western and Central Europe	1,210	1,140	1,290	0.4	0.4	0.4
Oceania	740	560	830	3.0	2.3	3.4
Global Estimate	**33,000**	**28,600**	**38,200**	**0.7**	**0.6**	**0.8**

Table 3.1 (Continued)

| Region or subregion | Opiates | | | | | |
| | Number (thousands) | | | Prevalence (percentage) | | |
	Best Estimate	Lower	Upper	Best Estimate	Lower	Upper
Africa	1,840	920	2,290	0.3	0.2	0.4
East Africa	220	160	310	0.1	0.1	0.2
North Africa	320	130	520	0.2	0.1	0.4
Southern Africa	290	200	310	0.3	0.2	0.4
West and Central Africa	1,000	430	1,140	0.4	0.2	0.5
Americas	1,620	1,430	1,800	0.3	0.2	0.3
Caribbean	80	50	160	0.3	0.2	0.6
Central America	20	20	20	0.1	0.1	0.1
North America	1,420	1,280	1,490	0.5	0.4	0.5
South America	110	90	120	0.04	0.03	0.05
Asia	9,860	7,480	12,990	0.3	0.3	0.5
Central Asia and Transcaucasia	440	420	450	0.8	0.8	0.8
East and South-East Asia	3,340	2,500	4,700	0.2	0.2	0.3
Near and Middle East/ South West Asia	3,320	2,410	4,440	1.2	0.9	1.6
South Asia	2,770	2,150	3,400	0.3	0.2	0.4
Europe	3,000	2,920	3,090	0.5	0.5	0.6
Eastern and South-Eastern Europe	1,890	1,880	1,890	0.8	0.8	0.8
Western and Central Europe	1,120	1,050	1,200	0.3	0.3	0.4
Oceania	40	40	60	0.2	0.2	0.2
Global Estimate	16,400	12,800	20,200	0.4	0.3	0.4

Table 3.2 Annual prevalence of the use of cocaine, amphetamines and "ecstasy," by region[3]

| Region or subregion | Cocaine | | | | | |
| | Number (thousands) | | | Prevalence (percentage) | | |
	Best Estimate	Lower	Upper	Best Estimate	Lower	Upper
Africa	2,590	800	4,680	0.4	0.1	0.8
East Africa	–	–	–	–	–	–
North Africa	30	30	40	0.02	0.02	0.03
Southern Africa	640	160	730	0.8	0.2	0.9
West and Central Africa	1,600	540	2,430	0.7	0.2	1.1
Americas	9,260	8,970	9,580	1.5	1.4	1.5
Caribbean	180	60	330	0.6	0.2	1.2
Central America	160	160	170	0.6	0.6	0.6
North America	5,580	5,460	5,690	1.8	1.7	1.8
South America	3,340	3,300	3,390	1.2	1.2	1.3
Asia	1,330	430	2,230	0.05	0.02	0.08
Central Asia and Trans-caucasia	–	–	–	–	–	–
East and South-East Asia	480	370	1,100	0.03	0.02	0.07
Near and Middle East/ South West Asia	90	50	140	0.03	0.02	0.05
South Asia	–	–	–	–	–	–
Europe	3,670	3,400	3,970	0.7	0.6	0.7
Eastern and South-Eastern Europe	540	290	810	0.2	0.1	0.4
Western and Central Europe	3,140	3,110	3,160	1.0	1.0	1.0
Oceania	380	380	460	1.5	1.5	1.9
Global Estimate	**17,200**	**14,000**	**20,900**	**0.4**	**0.3**	**0.4**

---

3 . Ibid. Annex I, p. XI.

Table 3.2 (Continued)

Region or subregion	ATS (amphetamine-type stimulant, excluding "ecstasy")					
	Number (thousands)			Prevalence (percentage)		
	Best Estimate	Lower	Upper	Best Estimate	Lower	Upper
Africa	5,200	1,360	8,950	0.9	0.2	1.5
East Africa	–	–	–	–	–	–
North Africa	740	260	1,220	0.6	0.2	0.9
Southern Africa	610	300	830	0.7	0.4	1.0
West and Central Africa	–	–	–	–	–	–
Americas	6,370	5,250	7,600	1.0	0.8	1.2
Caribbean	210	20	520	0.8	0.1	1.9
Central America	340	340	340	1.3	1.3	1.3
North America	4,410	3,710	5,100	1.4	1.2	1.6
South America	1,410	1,170	1,640	0.5	0.4	0.6
Asia	19,520	4,530	34,520	0.7	0.2	1.2
Central Asia and Trans-caucasia	–	–	–	–	–	–
East and South-East Asia	8,980	3,440	20,400	0.6	0.2	1.3
Near and Middle East/ South West Asia	440	370	820	0.2	0.1	0.3
South Asia	–	–	–	–	–	–
Europe	2,800	2,400	3,220	0.5	0.4	0.6
Eastern and South-Eastern Europe	850	470	1,230	0.4	0.2	0.5
Western and Central Europe	1,950	1,920	1,980	0.6	0.6	0.6
Oceania	510	410	530	2.1	1.7	2.2
Global Estimate	34,400	13,900	54,800	0.7	0.3	1.2

Continued ▶

Table 3.2 (Continued)

Region or subregion	"Ecstasy"					
	Number (thousands)			Prevalence (percentage)		
	Best Estimate	Lower	Upper	Best Estimate	Lower	Upper
Africa	1,080	350	1,880	0.2	0.1	0.3
East Africa	–	–	–	–	–	–
North Africa	–	–	–	–	–	–
Southern Africa	250	140	310	0.3	0.2	0.4
West and Central Africa	–	–	–	–	–	–
Americas	3,210	2,960	3,530	0.5	0.5	0.6
Caribbean	50	10	160	0.2	0.04	0.6
Central America	30	20	40	0.1	0.1	0.1
North America	2,770	2,740	2,800	0.9	0.9	0.9
South America	370	190	550	0.1	0.1	0.2
Asia	10,750	2,650	18,850	0.4	0.1	0.7
Central Asia and Trans-caucasia	–	–	–	–	–	–
East and South-East Asia	3,180	1,630	6,630	0.2	0.1	0.4
Near and Middle East/ South West Asia	–	–	–	–	–	–
South Asia	–	–	–	–	-	-
Europe	3,000	2,740	3,260	0.5	0.5	0.6
Eastern and South-Eastern Europe	1,340	1,110	1,580	0.6	0.5	0.7
Western and Central Europe	1,650	1,630	1,680	0.5	0.5	0.5
Oceania	720	700	720	2.9	2.9	2.9
Global Estimate	**18,800**	**28,200**	**9,400**	**0.4**	**0.2**	**0.6**

Psychoses are characterized by severe disorders of psychic functions and originate in the central nervous system. They affect the structural change of perception and experience and can be differentiated from other psychic disorders through symptoms and disease progression. One of the major psychoses is schizophrenia, a term established in 1911 by Swiss psychiatrist Paul Eugen Bleuler. The cause of schizophrenia is thought to be a metabolic dopamine disorder in the central nervous system. To this day, the exact emergence of this disease is not completely understood. There is evidence that somatic changes in the transmitter metabolism of the brain may play a crucial role in the psychological vulnerability of the affected person. Severe stress may trigger a psychotic episode, for example, the death of a close relative, relocation, health issues, or pregnancy. Genetic disposition is sometimes presumed. Children whose parents have schizophrenia are at a higher risk for developing schizophrenia compared with those who do not have a family history of the disorder. Approximately 1% of the population in Western countries has schizophrenia. Typically, schizophrenia initially manifests during late adolescence, but onset is possible at any time. Symptoms can include thought and speech disorders, illogical sentence structures, and predominantly perceptual disorders, such as hallucinations. Acoustic and visual hallucinations are some of the main symptoms of schizophrenia. Other indications of possible schizophrenia include hearing voices, being controlled by others, being manipulated from the outside, and following the orders of higher powers. Karl Jaspers postulated three criteria for delusions:

1. Absolute subjective certainty.
2. Incorrectability.
3. Impossibility of content.

These criteria still apply. Other symptoms of schizophrenia include the freezing of motion and speech. Catatonia is the abnormally extended arrest in a certain position. It is one of the indications of catatonic schizophrenia. The diagnosis of schizophrenia is based on the recognition of symptoms. Patients with the disorder must take long-term medications, possibly for the rest of their lives. Patients may become incompliant with their medications and feel as though they are "better" and choose to discontinue their medications, at which time they may have a relapse and, thus, have misjudged the scope of the disease. To this end, long-term injectable forms of effective drugs for the treatment of schizophrenia may help alleviate issues of patient adherence. A patient's trust in his or her physician is also of the utmost importance in such cases.

Affective disorders are characterized mainly by mood changes. We differentiate between two basic types of mood disorders, depression and manic depression (bipolar disorder), which includes symptoms of both stages. Classification is descriptive because the causes of affective disorders have not yet been clarified. Many scientists favor a genetic component in cases of mania rather than in cases of endogenous depression. In cases of depression, we must differentiate between the basic endogenous depression and depressive disorder, or reactive depression. Basic (endogenous) depression is the most frequent type of psychic disorder, with women affected twice as often as men. Significant emotional, social, or job-related factors may trigger depressive conditions. Severe organic diseases, such as tumors, Cushing's disease, brain tumors, or multiple sclerosis, may also trigger depression. Medications such as β-blockers or cytostatics may also cause depression. Diagnosis is based on patient history, clinical examination, and medical consultation. Medication compliance varies. Those who experience an acute manic episode may be driven and have flights of ideas. They may sleep little and make nonsensical decisions, but they may also lack the realization that they are ill and sensible communication may be impossible. Neuroleptics and sedatives may be indicated during the acute manic stage. During the depressive stage, SSRIs may be indicated because this affective disorder is thought to be caused by an imbalance of the neurotransmitters serotonin and norepinephrine in the central nervous system. Additional antidepressants include MOAs and tricyclic antidepressants. In cases of bipolar affective disorders, lithium is sometimes prescribed. In some cases, antidepressants, lithium, and mood stabilizers, such as lamotrigine, valproic acid, and carbamazepine, can be used as a long-term prophylaxis of attacks for some patients with affective disorders.

Eating disorders, such as anorexia nervosa and bulimia, are sometimes seen in young people. These disorders also belong to the fields of psychiatry, psychosomatics, and psychotherapy.

Typical characteristics of neuroses include anxiety disorders, obsessive-compulsive disorders, and somatoform disorders (previously termed "hysteria"). These, like many personality disorders, are typically treated with psychotherapy and form the core of psychosomatic medicine.

Geriatric psychiatry addresses psychiatric diseases in those of older age and include disorders such as dementia, which is increasing in prevalence, likely due to the fact that our lifespan is much longer today than it was in the past. In the foreseeable future, prevalence of Alzheimer's disease will be 10%. This is of considerable consequence for a national economy.

Another growing field of psychiatry is pediatric psychiatry. Our modern lifestyle, which is often characterized by stress, the everyday "rush," overstimulation, neglect, and the lack of parental care, may cause alienation of children from family, security, love, discipline, and values of tolerance.

The broad range of forensic psychiatry is most certainly challenging and fascinating. Movies like *The Silence of the Lambs* have given us dramatic (albeit fictional) and sensational insights into the world of the psychopathologically deranged and their extreme acts of violence. Violence is not limited to brutal physical violence but can include sexual and aggressive assaults on women, men, and children. Currently, therapeutic options are relatively limited in forensic psychiatry. With the exception of lifetime institutionalization in a psychiatric facility and long-term medication, there are very limited psychotherapeutic approaches. It is risky for any psychiatrist or reviewer to venture a prognosis for such a patient. Falsely presumed improvement may lead to the discharge of the patient, even if only for hours, during which the psychologically ill person may commit further crimes. Great responsibility weighs heavily on the psychiatric reviewer. As a consequence, he or she may be overly strict in order to protect themselves or, in order to avoid this, they may quickly assume improvement that could only be simulated.

We must ask ourselves, generally speaking, whether psychotherapy can be effective in the context of pressure to adapt within a closed facility. Furthermore, we must realize that illness and diseases are subject to cultural distinctions. In the United States, we may consider something to be an illness or disease that is viewed as being normal in another country. The converse is also true. Traditionally, alcohol consumption is tolerated in Western countries. By contrast, in many Islamic countries, alcohol consumption is prohibited and at times avenged. Malarial anemia is considered common in some parts of Africa. Morbid obesity, a spreading condition in Western countries, is largely unknown to North Koreans. Thus, as we can see, pathology defines diseases and their courses, but the ways in which we view these diseases is subject to cultural variations.

3.13 Surgery

Surgery is undoubtedly one of the most fascinating and exciting specialty areas in medicine. The segmentation of this field creates a broad scope of opportunities. A student can be ensured a fulfilling career as a surgeon only if he or she thoroughly studies theory, is in good health, makes considerable effort, and is manually dexterous. Similar to internal medicine, postgraduate training regulations in surgery are constantly changing. Currently, postgraduate training for surgeons in Germany lasts six years and may be followed by advanced training for vascular or pediatric surgery. Other Western countries may require basic postgraduate surgical training of two years followed by advanced training for the subspecialty areas of thoracic or cardiac surgery. Similar to those in internal medicine, discussions take place about, for example, why a young physician must learn how to perform surgery on the ankle joint if he or she really wants to become a cardiac surgeon and will never operate on an ankle again. In the context of decreasing resources in the health care system and the increasing number of liability lawsuits, appropriateness of Western postgraduate training regulation has been under close scrutiny. For example, in the Netherlands, postgraduate training lasts six years. Within this time, the physician must go through different subspecialty areas lasting three months each. The cycle starts in the polyclinic, continues in trauma surgery, oncology, anesthesiology, and ends in the polyclinic. The cycle then continues through general surgery, oncology, vascular surgery, and returns to the polyclinic. From here it starts all over again. The goal is that the surgeon-to-be spends at least one year in every field of surgery. In other places, the duration of each stage is six months instead of three, because three months at one time is considered insufficient. I believe that it is important to complete an internship in every field of surgery. It is helpful to have assisted in a cardiac intervention, even for someone who wants to become a plastic surgeon, just as it is important for a surgeon performing research to have assisted in thoracic surgeries. In addition, sometimes each subspecialty area can only be found in a small number of specialty clinics. We learned about this situation in Section 3.8 "Internal Medicine." Large clinics that focus on endocrine surgeries cannot offer sufficient teaching surgeries for thoracic or plastic interventions. In transplantation centers, which may perform 50 to 100 kidney or liver transplantations per year, not enough tumor surgeries can be performed to train young interns. Therefore, it is important to perform such training in a large clinic, but it is as important to change clinical settings during training. Moreover, we have learned that smoking and obesity pose risks to our health, but so does the surgeon. Various international double-blind studies have proven that postoperative outcomes are better and postoperative complications are fewer if the performing surgeon has focused on a limited number of surgery types.

Most surgeons focus on a particular field, including the following:

- Abdominal surgery.
- Heart surgery.
- Vascular surgery.
- Thoracic surgery.
- Pediatric surgery.
- Plastic surgery.

For forensic reasons alone it is no longer acceptable to be active in two or more fields. In this context, it should be noted that the majority of liability lawsuits in Western countries are filed in the areas of orthopaedics, trauma surgery, and gynecology.

Generally, we differentiate between general and specialized surgery. In general surgery, the physician learns surgical techniques, including biopsies, catheter and tube placement, as well as the basics of asepsis and antisepsis, preoperative diagnostics—which is usually performed by internists and radiologists—and postoperative therapy. Postoperative therapy includes nutrition, pain therapy, monitoring and adjusting electrolyte and acid–base balances, intravenous therapy, and the understanding and techniques of blood transfusion and coagulation.

Blood transfusion and coagulation are topics of growing importance. Blood transfusions are subject to increasing regulatory requirements. In addition, in clinical surgery procedures, we have learned that it does not always make sense, for example, for the anesthesiologist to infuse stored blood at one end of the operating table while blood is removed by suction and discarded at the injury site during surgery of a patient with injured pelvic veins. Blood-conserving surgeries are on the rise. Here, blood is suctioned, immediately purified, and transfused back into the same patient. For logistical reasons it is sometimes not possible to provide sufficient units of blood during such a short period of time. This is the case in major surgeries, such as liver or spleen ruptures. Considerate handling of banked blood is an absolute priority. The phlebotomist responsible for transfusions works closely with the surgeon and must possess considerable logistic abilities, including establishing quick contact with various blood banks if not enough units of a particular blood type are available on site, reliable blood typing, and taking into account the effects of mass transfusions. The clinical picture of coagulation disorders, such as disseminated intravascular coagulation, thrombocytopenia, various rare antibodies, such as warm and cold agglutinins, is highly interesting and a frequent subject of research projects. The life of a patient is in acute danger if coagulation problems occur.

Every physician should be able to suture the skin. Treatment and healing of wounds and local and conductive anesthesia are part of general surgery. The indications for surgery and medico-legal issues are of growing importance and pose new challenges for the physician. In general, it is true that the correct indication is the key to a successful surgery. In microbiology and hygiene, we were introduced to infections caused while staying in the hospital, such as "hospitalism" and nosocomial infection. Another central focus of surgery is oncologic surgery, including tumor treatment in collaboration with radiotherapy, chemotherapy, and postoperative care. The application of compression dressings, the use of physical therapy, and medical assessment are all part of general surgery. Ultrasonography may be part of surgery, internal medicine, or X-ray diagnostics, depending on country and clinic. Endoscopy belongs to the field of surgery. In some clinics, it is moved into its own department and is carried out by internists. Never ending discussions about the correct way to perform endoscopy have not produced the silver bullet. I have met great surgeons who did an excellent job with endoscopies. An inexperienced internist is likely to do more harm than good.

3.13.1 Abdominal Surgery

The therapeutic spectrum of abdominal surgery contains diseases of the gastrointestinal tract, from the esophagus to anus, internal organs, and the thyroid, parathyroid, and adrenal glands. In some clinics, diseases of the breast are covered by general surgery, but, in the majority of Europe, breast surgery is an established part of gynecology. As in many other areas, countries and medical schools ultimately determine if breast surgery is part of general surgery or gynecology. There are 170 types of abdominal surgery, many of which involve the stomach, gallbladder, and intestines (called major surgeries). During postgraduate training, specialists are likely to perform 100 smaller surgeries, including appendectomy, varicocele repair, hernia surgery, artificial anus sphincter implantation, and vascular and nerve sutures.

The most frequent indication in thyroid diseases is nodular or multinodular goiter. Thyroid tumors are another indication for thyroid surgery. In particular, anaplastic carcinoma is a fast-growing, extremely aggressive type of tumor. Modern surgical procedures include medial neck incision and neuromonitoring. Recurrent lesions should be avoided as much as possible. Dialysis for kidney diseases has resulted in an increasing incidence of secondary and tertiary hyperparathyroidism and a rising number of parathyroid surgeries within the last 30 years. Significant experience and skill are required to recognize and resect the parathyroid glands. Adrenal resection is performed primarily in patients with Conn's syndrome and Cushing's syndrome as well as in those with pheochromocytoma. These surgical procedures are generally performed in large clinics and require postoperative adrenocorticosteroid substitution for the rest of the patient's life.

In the area of the upper gastrointestinal tract, the incidence of esophageal carcinoma has dramatically increased without any distinct cause. Esophageal varices following portal hypertension and esophageal rupture are rare but dreaded conditions (**Fig. 3.20**). As with other major surgeries, performing esophageal resection requires years of training and experience. It is rated to be at the highest level of surgical difficulty.

Gastric cancer is the main indication for surgeries of the stomach. The incidence of gastric cancer is higher in Japan than in Europe. Correlation to nutrition has been researched but not clarified. In gastric cancer, lymphogenic metastasis occurs early on. Surgery is indicated if distant metastases are not present; if they are present, palliative tubing is indicated while surgery is not. Similar to other medical fields, therapy must be individualized depending on the type of tumor. Not every gastric cancer can or should be surgically treated. Instead, the tumor review board, including the oncologist, pathologist, and radiologist, is likely to define the best treatment for the patient. There is no standard recommendation for the various gastric resections. The physician should follow the recommendations and clinical practice guidelines of major professional medical organizations.

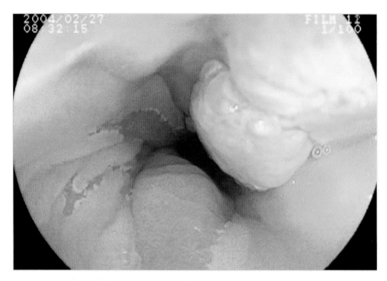

Fig. 3.20 Esophageal adenocarcinoma with stenosis.

Lately, bariatric surgery has become a much-discussed topic. Partial resection of the stomach, performed by laparoscopy, allows patients only small amounts of food intake. The production site of the peptide hormone ghrelin, which is located in the fundus of the stomach, is also resected. This procedure inhibits intense feelings of hunger. The indication for this procedure is certainly controversial because a healthy organ is partially removed. Once again, medicine finds itself knee-deep in ethical dilemmas and the years to come may help shed light on the best route to take.

Diagnosis and therapy of anal diseases and colorectal cancer—the third most common type of cancer in US males and females, the second most common type of cancer in German females and third most common type of cancer in German males—belong to the area of the lower gastrointestinal tract.

Pancreatic surgery and duodenum-preserving pancreatic head resection are usually lumped together as pancreatogenic surgery. This type of surgery is also extremely difficult and should only be performed by skilled surgeons. Similar to gastric cancer, pancreatic cancer is an unwelcome diagnosis as its survival rates are low because it metastasizes early and is an extremely aggressive carcinoma.

Liver surgery is another subspecialty of abdominal surgery. Common liver surgeries include liver cysts and tumor resections and liver transplantations. The field of general surgery is an example of how we build on the knowledge imparted in anatomy and histology. Histology taught us the structure of the liver and its accompanying sinusoids. We learned about the periportal region and what the histologic section of a liver cell (including azan staining) looks like. We developed a feeling for tissues and will apply this knowledge in the area of liver surgery. In pathology, we learned about conditions such as liver tumors, liver disorders, inflammation, and micro- and macronodular cirrhosis. In embryology, we studied the liver and pancreas and understood what is meant by annular pancreas and why there was a blood-forming embryonic stage in the spleen and the liver. Particularly for the fields of surgery and internal medicine, knowledge is structured like a puzzle. This makes us realize the true value of the knowledge we gain from preclinical studies.

3.13.2 Heart Surgery

In open-heart surgeries, patients are connected to a heart–lung machine. Surgeries without the heart–lung machine include interventions at the ductus arteriosus, and coarctation of the aorta. Surgeries that require the heart–lung machine include thoracic aortic aneurysms, valve defects, coronary heart diseases, and congenital heart defects. Heart surgery is a very emotional issue in public view. The surgeon must be extremely knowledgeable about cardiac anatomy and physiology and possess a high level of surgical experience. Congenital heart defects, pulmonary stenosis, and aortic insufficiency are discussed as part of internal medicine and are treated as part of heart surgery. Endoscopic valve surgeries, particularly in cases of mitral valve defects, are ground-breaking developments in heart surgery.

Coronary artery bypass graft surgery is the most common cardiac intervention. In arteriosclerotic occlusion of the coronary arteries the bypass is placed between the aorta and coronary artery (**Fig. 3.21**). Pacemaker implantation, cardiac trauma care, and the treatment of pericardial diseases also belong to the field of heart surgery. Heart surgery is an interesting and highly complex specialty, usually found in major clinics with an affiliated cardiology department. Heart surgeons are generally absorbed by their work and left with very little private time. Those who like being at the center of a medical specialty that is at the center of attention feel comfortable with heart surgery. Public and media interest is very much focused on the areas of cardiology, transplantation surgery, oncologic surgery, and heart surgery. But one also must consider that a heart surgeon is likely to be tied to a clinic for the rest of his life and unlikely to set up a private practice. Cardiac surgery requires long hours and many years of hard work, especially when some surgeries last 6 hours or more and pose excessive physical strain on the surgeon. If the medical student does not mind all these aspects, heart surgery may be his vocation.

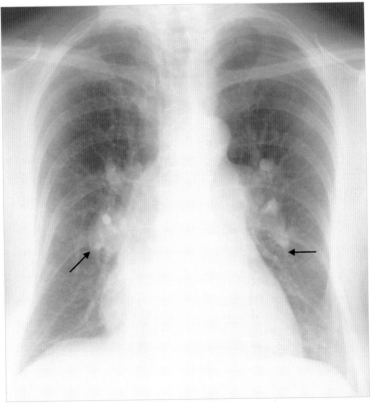

Fig. 3.21 A 75-year-old woman with coronary heart disease and status post–aortocoronary venous bypass. Central vessels are thickened with a significant mismatch between the segmental arteries and accompanying bronchi and an abrupt reduction in caliber toward the periphery (arrows).

3.13.3 Vascular Surgery

Socioeconomic lifestyle factors, such as obesity, lack of exercise, or smoking, may cause vascular occlusions, particularly of the lower extremities. Vascular surgery is a most interesting and challenging field that demands that the surgeon has a high level of dexterity and stamina. In major clinics specializing in vascular surgery, it is possible that only a few surgeries are conducted each day because these interventions can last for hours. Some of the most common procedures in vascular surgery include traditional bypasses in the lower extremities, carotid surgery, and aneurysm repair. Endovascular procedures are becoming increasingly popular. They also should take place in special clinics. We can consider vascular surgery to be a traditional craft. The surgeon must expose vessels for hours, suture anastomoses, and test if the anastomoses are still conducting or already thrombotic. Whoever is eager to progress quickly in vascular surgery should begin practicing vascular surgery on animals. By operating on the abdominal aorta of pigs or microscopic anastomoses in rats, physicians learn the techniques that they will need every day in vascular surgery. In vascular surgery especially, but also in general and trauma surgery, the difference between theorists and pragmatists becomes apparent. True surgeons are those who can handle an abdominal aneurysm or complicated stomach bleeding at night during their emergency service.

3.13.4 Thoracic Surgery

Thoracic surgery includes thoracic trauma, surgical correction of funnel chests, and resection of pulmonary metastases in bronchial cancer. Ultimately, lung cancer is primarily the domain of radiology. Thoracic surgery also includes the surgical correction of pulmonary malformation, cysts, and emphysema, as well as inflammatory pulmonary diseases with abscesses and the surgical treatment of tubercular lesions. Video-assisted thoracoscopic surgery (VATS) has become a popular technique in this surgical field.

Successful thoracic surgery requires an understanding of anatomic structures in order to deduce the topographic relations of the organs. Structures located in the thorax, such as the lungs, mediastinum, the heart muscle and the pericardium, and the sensitive motor lymph vessels—in particular, the thoracic duct—are very fragile and must not be damaged during surgery. The same is true for the gaseous exchange in the lungs that we learned about in physiology and the causative pathophysiologic processes taking place in cases of emphysema, atelectasis, or tension pneumothorax. Diagnostics applied in thoracic surgery include conventional lung X-rays, MRI, rigid or flexible bronchoscopy, and evermore relevant thoracoscopy.

Complications of a thoracic trauma include injuries involving costal vessel bleeding in cases of multiple rib fractures and the filling of the lung alveoli with liquid, be it blood, interstitial fluid, or lymph. In either case, gaseous exchange is considerably inhibited, which causes—depending on the extent of alveolar congestion—hypoxia in addition to the existing trauma or blood loss. Dyspnea is a common symptom in thoracic trauma. Rapid intervention that involves eliminating the cause and intubating the patient is the therapy of choice. Cricothyrotomy is a frequent subject of discussion in thoracic surgery as well as in emergency medicine. Here, as in many medical fields, there are different mindsets. I know of emergency physicians who have never performed cricothyrotomy (puncture into the ligament between the thyroid cartilage and the cricoid cartilage to ventilate the patient) to insert a breathing tube.

Lung resection procedures vary, but they all focus on the affected pulmonary lobe. In atelectasis, tumors, or thoracic injuries, the tumorally affected or traumatized parts of the lung must be resected. Thoracic surgery addresses resection of pulmonary lobes, or the entire lung, as well as congenital lung diseases, such as bronchial stenosis, bronchogenic cysts, and others. Indications for lung transplantation include cystic fibrosis, COPD, primary pulmonary hypertension, and, according to the New York Heart Association, Eisenmenger's syndrome.

3.13.5 Pediatric Surgery

Pediatric surgery involves the diagnosis and surgical treatment of diseases during childhood. Every surgeon who has opened the abdomen of a child with suspected appendicitis and found black intestines with a foul odor knows the complications lurking behind a seemingly normal finding of acute appendicitis. The broad spectrum of pediatric surgery includes common appendicitis, abdominal tumors, as well as difficult-to-diagnose conditions such as ileus and volvulus. Common diseases include Hirschsprung's disease, aganglionosis with mega rectum, invagination, intestinal atresia, and Meckel's diverticulum. In pediatric surgery, the instruments used are smaller than those used in adult surgeries. Complications are different and much more severe than in surgeries on adults. One of the most frequent cases in pediatric surgery is inguinal hernia. Caused by the low surfactant concentration in the lungs, the newborn or premature infant breathes harder and produces increased pressure onto the inguinal canal, which can result in bilateral inguinal hernia. In some countries, urologic surgery, including urachal fistula, urethral atresia, and incontinence improvement, is performed by pediatric surgeons. Those who enjoy working with children, and who also wish to practice in a very interesting and challenging field with increasing responsibility, may feel at home with pediatric surgery.

3.13.6 Plastic Surgery

Plastic and reconstructive surgery is a department frequently located in large hospitals and is sometimes combined with burn centers. Plastic surgery includes reconstruction after severe burns with skin grafts, reconstructive flap surgery—particularly mastectomy—or reconstructive procedures following radiation with ensuing skin ulceration (**Fig. 3.22**). Plastic surgery is frequently performed under the microscope. The surgeon must be able to concentrate, be calm and enjoy working accurately to the millimeter. Areas that require specialized departments include the reconstruction of facial nerves in combination with oral and maxillofacial surgery, otoplasty of protruding ears (ear pinning) in children, and breast reconstruction.

Plastic and reconstructive surgery is an important medical field. However, some physicians who choose this specialty do not work in plastic and reconstructive surgery but exclusively in cosmetic surgery.

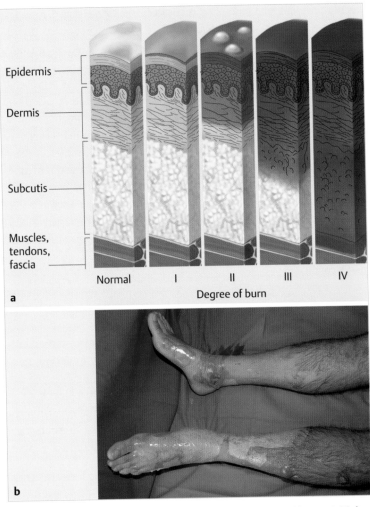

Fig. 3.22 Degree of burn. **a** Classification according to depth of burn (degrees I–IV). **b** Third degree burns of both feet at transition to lower calf with second degree (blister formation).

In the area of plastic surgery it is obvious that every surgical activity requires a sense and feeling for tissues. In the surgical field, there are two aspects that must be observed. The surgeon must properly communicate with the patient. He or she must explain the surgery in a way that the patient understands and is able to give informed consent. The patient delivers information about their condition and disease stage by the way they enter the room or lie in bed during rounds. The patient may smile, be focused, oriented, euphoric, depressed, or their face may be distorted with pain. This impression registers with the physician and provides him or her with crucial information about the patient. The same applies to tissues. Once a surgeon has sutured a nerve with a 5-0 suture, they know the delicacy of this procedure and that they can only conduct it wearing magnifying spectacles or under the microscope. Once the surgeon has seen the rupture of the lesser trochanter at the femur, they know that it requires stabilization to reset this osseous structure because it is of major importance for muscle insertion. When removing an ingrown intramedullary nail from the osseous tissue, the surgeon must use a hammer like a steel worker. Plastic surgery reveals the surgeon's sensitivity to delicate structures, their ability to suture a bleeding vascular anastomotic insufficiency, and to remain calm and focused when they encounter difficult tissue conditions.

3.14 Anesthesia, Emergency Medicine, and Pain Medicine

On October 16, 1846, the first successful case of anesthesia during surgery was demonstrated at the Massachusetts General Hospital. Since that day, anesthesia has undergone fundamental changes and developments.

Increasing numbers of surgeries can be conducted on increasingly younger patients. For example, surgeries on newborns with a deformity of the abdominal wall are not uncommon. Even patients of 100 years of age can be anesthetized using today's modern medicine, for example, during hip replacement surgery. Anesthesiologic therapies include inhalation anesthetics, analgesics and muscle relaxants, intravenous hypnotics, and sedatives. Thorough knowledge of physiology, biochemistry, and pharmacology are foundations for the successful anesthesiologist. Anesthesia requires special attention in cardiac surgeries or surgeries of newborns, and the field has become an intellectually demanding modern specialty. Anesthesiologists decide whether a patient can undergo surgery and what type of anesthetic will be provided. In some cases, it may be their decision as to whether a patient is moved to the intensive care unit and for how long they must remain there. Few hospitals are likely to have both a dermatology and ophthalmology department, but every surgical specialty requires its own anesthesiology department. Anesthesiology is an option for a part-time career or for resident physicians to work in hospitals or large emergency centers.

A prerequisite for every anesthesiologist—actually for every physician—is the ability to intubate a patient. The modern-day anesthesiologist faces challenges, such as difficult respiratory passages in patients with a pyknic physique, malignant hyperthermia (rare), or allergic reactions to drugs.

Today's anesthesiologist has become a medical economist. He or she must be proficient in pain therapy, intensive care, and logistic issues. But beyond medical competence, organizational talent is required. The anesthesiologist can be in charge of scheduling surgeries, organizing the recovery room, intensive care unit, outpatient pain management, as well as planning and organizing the anesthesia care team when a severely injured person is admitted. Anesthesia is the right career for someone who feels a calling for the above-mentioned activities, is a good organizer, wants to interface with surgery and diagnostics, and is willing to accept considerable responsibility for patients.

Emergency medicine and anesthesiologic intensive care primarily address cardiovascular emergencies. These include cardiac infarction, pulmonary embolism, hypertension, cardiogenic shock, and all other shock conditions. Another group of disorders addressed by emergency medicine is respiratory disease, such as bronchial asthma and laryngeal edema. Intoxications make up the next group of conditions dealt with by emergency medicine physicians. We learned about poisonings in pharmacology and will face the lethal consequences in forensic medicine. Drug consumption fueled by the overabundance of designer drugs is the most common cause of intoxication. Next on the list of intoxications is alcohol intoxication. Mushroom poisonings happen rather infrequently. Often no antidote exists and the condition must be treated symptomatically, which means vital functions must be stabilized. Every physician should know emergency medicine, particularly how to diagnosis and provide therapy for acutely life-threatening cardiovascular and pulmonary conditions. Physicians must also master the small number of common emergencies in pediatrics, otolaryngology, ophthalmology, urology, and neurology. In some European countries, emergency medicine still requires additional training. In the United States, the emergency physician is usually the one heading the emergency department. Emergency physicians are health care professionals able to act quickly in distress, such as in cases of burns, mentally and emotionally exceptional situations, motor vehicle collisions, or respiratory distress in a pediatric patient. They must intuitively decide without hesitation what treatment to choose. The pragmatic person who is able to help in the ambulance, helicopter, or emergency department may find his calling in this specialty.

Pain therapy has undergone tremendous development during the past few decades. This development includes all related aspects, such as our understanding of pain, knowledge of the various receptors in the central nervous system, and pain medication like opioids and their derivatives. The pain therapist must have thorough experience and knowledge of the physiologic basics of pain and the existing pain pathways. They must approach their patients with empathy, understanding, and compassion. They must *listen* to the patient. A surgeon is not likely to have the same amount of time to communicate with their patients as the pain specialist, so diagnostics and treatment decisions may rely heavily on the one-on-one communication between patient and pain specialist. It is true that pain medication is a multibillion-dollar industry, and the trend is rising. Every year, the pharmaceutical industry brings new pain medications to the market. Pain management in patients with cancer is one of the central tasks in pain departments due to increasing life expectancy and the incidence of oncologic diseases. Other common ailments treated by pain therapists are chronic headache and back pain. Concomitant complaints, such as nausea and somnolence, are also treated. A common class of pain medications called nonsteroidal anti-inflammatory drugs contributes to the pathogenesis of gastric ulcers if taken over long periods of time, so pain therapists must counsel their patients to take these pain medications with food as the stomach mucosa must be protected from developing such ulcers.

At this point, I would like to mention anesthesia and intensive care medicine. In recent years, this specialty, along with emergency medicine, has improved the reputation of the anesthesiologist within the field of medicine. Anesthesia and intensive care includes procedures such as introducing a central venous catheter line, arterial cannula, punctures, bronchoscopy, and tracheotomy.

Pain therapy is a perfect specialty for physicians who possess the necessary psychological sensibility to work and communicate with patients in physical pain. Highly potent analgesics are part of this therapy. The pain therapist must be thoroughly knowledgeable about the effects of all analgesics and find the proper dosage for every patient. This is an interesting challenge in a medical field with plenty of prospects for everyone who possesses sound knowledge of all aspects pertaining to pain therapy.

3.15 Orthopaedic and Trauma Surgery

In Germany, as in other places, the separate fields of orthopaedics and trauma surgery have now mostly merged into a single specialty. The creation of a specialist in orthopaedic and trauma surgery aligns with that of English-speaking countries, which do not differentiate between orthopaedic and trauma surgery.

The average life expectancy among most citizens of the Western world is 75 years or older, which also means that degenerative diseases are on the rise. At the same time, people have growing expectations with regard to their mobility and independence. Therefore, orthopaedic surgery is of growing importance, particularly in the realm of prosthetics. In Germany, 11,649 shoulder, 143,024 knee, and 210,384 hip replacements are carried out each year (DESTATIS 2013). According to the Agency for Healthcare Research and Quality, about 53,000 people in the United States have shoulder replacement surgery every year, and more than 900,000 have knee and hip replacement surgery (AHRQ 2014). Thanks to improvements in implantation and surgical techniques, the average lifetime of more than 90% of prostheses is 15 years. A considerable part of this success is owed to postoperative rehabilitation, without which the functionality of joints could not be restored to this extent (**Fig. 3.23**).

Another large area of orthopaedics involves the spine. Within different medical societies, different schools of thought have emerged. In Western countries, spine surgery—particularly surgery of the intervertebral disks—is divided between orthopaedics and neurosurgery. (However, there has been no final decision as to whether spine surgery belongs to orthopaedics or neurosurgery.) The subspecialty also shows the number of surgical interventions is growing, which is particularly true for surgeries of the intervertebral disks and in cases of spinal canal stenosis. The reason for the increased incidence is thought to be related to demographic development. Surgery is indicated in cases of pain and neurologic deficits, although an exact diagnosis generally requires MRI.

This specialty area includes endoprosthetics and spine surgery, as mentioned above, but also interdisciplinary challenges, such as congenital skeletal deformation in children, within the scope of pediatric orthopaedics, hand surgery—for example, carpal tunnel syndrome, Dupuytren's contracture—misalignment after injuries, and soft-tissue and bone cancer surgeries.

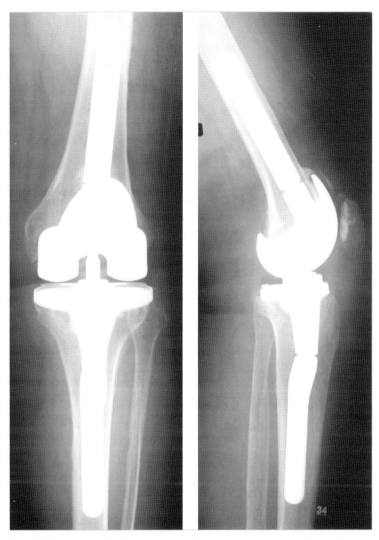

Fig. 3.23 Radiographs of a fistulous periprosthetic infection after a prosthesis of the knee joint had been exchanged and multiple soft-tissue revisions had been performed.

Another part of this new specialty involves the entire surgical range of trauma-related injury. Treatment options have also improved in this field, due in part to new implants, such as fixed-angle plate systems, and minimally invasive surgical procedures. At the same time, methods and procedures—so-called trauma management—have changed. Trauma centers execute standardized procedures for their patients comparable to the procedures for stroke or cardiac infarctions. These standards include options for intensive care, surgical procedures, interdisciplinary treatment (e.g., for thoracic, abdominal, urologic injuries), as well as criteria for relocating patients to specialized facilities (e.g., head injuries, paraplegic symptoms, severe burns).

All in all, orthopaedics and trauma surgery form a huge field in medicine and are particularly attractive due to the abundance of subspecialties. Thorough knowledge of anatomy, dexterity, and the enjoyment of manual skills and work are mandatory. However, no other specialty area exists with a comparable number of (successful) lawsuits. The patients in question usually refer to a long disease history and expect complete restoration of all malfunctions and freedom from symptoms. Against this backdrop, it is mandatory to provide and document the differential diagnosis. The patient must be able to give informed consent—and that consent thoroughly documented—and they must be made aware and understand all of their alternative treatment options (conservative vs. surgical therapy) and their associated risks. Expectations and demands of the patients must be taken into account.

3.16 Urology

In medieval times, barber surgeons who specialized in cataract treatments were infamous at fairs, as were stone cutters who brutally performed urethral dilatation after syphilitic infections or urinary stone extractions without the use of any sterile equipment or the use of anesthesia. Fortunately, modern urology has changed. As in most other medical specialties, knowledge of anatomy and embryology is essential for diagnosing urological diseases. Urology is an interesting interdisciplinary medical field due to the close collaboration with other specialties, such as nephrology, gynecology, dermatology, surgery, X-ray diagnostics, and bacteriology. A clinical examination in urology involves an examination of male and female genitals, prostate palpation, and tapping of the renal bed (**Fig. 3.24**). Ultrasonography is an important diagnostic tool in urology. Modern diagnostics without the use of ultrasonography to visualize the kidneys, bladder, and the prostate is inconceivable. Therefore, thorough knowledge of ultrasonography is mandatory for practicing this specialty. Other diagnostics may include angiography, CT, and MRI for depicting the

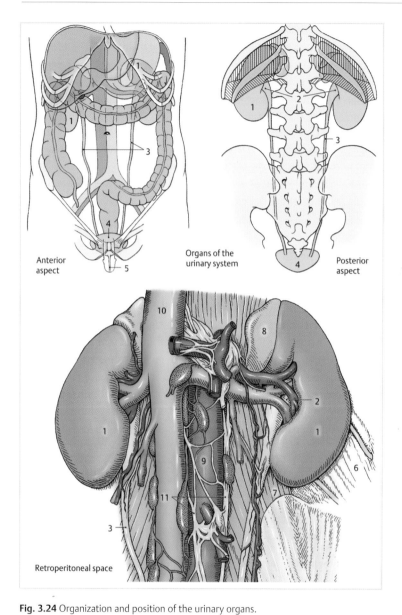

Fig. 3.24 Organization and position of the urinary organs.
1 Kidneys, 2 Renal pelves, 3 Ureters, 4 Urinary bladder, 5 Urethra, 6 Quadratus lumborum muscle, 7 Psoas major muscle, 8 Adrenal glands, 9 Aorta, 10 Inferior vena cava, 11 Sympathetic trunk

ureters, expanded renal pelves, or in cases of renal parenchyma; conventional X-ray may be used for investigative urography using radiocontrast agents. Special examinations include voiding cystourethrogram in order to clarify if physiologic micturition is possible and phlebography (or cardiograph) in order to depict the vessels of the male genitals. Furthermore, urologic diagnostics include endoscopy with cystoscopy and percutaneous nephroscopy, which is the percutaneous examination of the renal tissue. Additional special examinations include biopsy procedures and urodynamic procedures, such as cytometry and urometry, which measure the pressure in ureter or bladder. As we can see, urologic diagnostics covers a large area and is a vital part of specialty training of urologists.

One of the cardinal symptoms of urologic disorders is a change in urine volume and quality. Oliguria is urine production of less than 500 mL in 24 hours. Polyuria is urine production of more than 4,000 mL in 24 hours. These symptoms are important parameters for the physician. Urinary tract infections, blood present in the urine, or renal pain with colicky radiation into the groin, as well as the symptoms of bladder infection, are some of the common complaints of patients with urologic conditions. Bladder infections are some of the most commonly seen postoperative complications and must be recognized (e.g., scrotal swelling and voiding disorders in cases of cancer).

In the area of nephrology and dialysis, physicians must collaborate with internists. Diseases that internists and urologists must both be familiar with and able to treat include renal tubular acidosis, renal insufficiency—particularly acute renal failure with hyperhydration and hyperkalemia—chronic renal insufficiency with arterial hypertension, and uremia. Every urologist must also be capable of treating renal hypertension and hypertensive heart conditions following kidney transplantations.

Urologic diagnostics and therapy depend on the anatomic structures of the human body. Renal diseases are caused by malformations or inflammatory conditions such as pyelonephritis, urosepsis, and interstitial nephritis. Tumors and renal stones are other areas of urologic intervention. Renal stones can be found along the entire urogenital tract, not exclusively in the renal pelvis.

With regard to diseases of the ureter and bladder, congenital malformations must first be noted. Chronic cystitis and injuries to the bladder and ureter following severe pelvic fractures must be urologically treated. Incidences of bladder cancer are less frequent than prostate cancer. In the Western world, prostate cancer is the most frequent type of cancer in males. More than 90% of males older than 80 years of age may become affected, and, unfortunately, the cause of prostate cancer is currently unknown. Usually, it presents as adenocarcinoma. Cancer therapy for this type of carcinoma has fundamentally changed in recent years. Urology also covers aspects such as diseases of the external genitals, andrology (more commonly known simply as men's health), fertility counseling, and erectile dysfunction.

The catalogs of required surgeries for urologists differ from country to country. In accordance with the guidelines of German medical associations, during specialty training, the aspiring urologist should perform an average of 50 kidney and ureter surgeries, 25 bladder surgeries, 25 prostate surgeries, and the same number of penile and external genital surgeries. In the United States, residents are required to achieve the number of procedures determined by the Accreditation Council for Graduate Medical Education (ACGME).[4]

Depending on the country, venereology, which is the diagnosis and therapy of sexually transmitted infections, belongs either to dermatology or urology. Typical sexually transmitted infections treated with penicillin include gonorrhea (an infection of the genitals caused by *Neisseria gonorrhoeae*), and syphilis (caused by *Treponema pallidum*). Sexually acquired infections also include the following:

- Chancroid (caused by *Haemophilus ducreyi*).
- Lymphogranuloma venereum, caused by *Chlamydia trachomatis*, responds well to macrolide antibiotics such as erythromycin. Chlamydial infections are ideally treated with tetracyclines or gyrase inhibitors such as ofloxacin.
- HIV/AIDS.
- Genital warts (condylomata acuminata).
- Mycoplasma genitalium infection.

Urology is a combination of diagnostics and therapy of the urogenital tract of both sexes. The urologist treats different disorders in different groups of patients, including children with hypospadias or epispadia, older men with prostate cancer or prostate hyperplasia, sexual dysfunction in men, or follow-up therapy for those who have undergone kidney transplantation. Urology is a welcome challenge to those looking for a

---

4 See http://www.acgme.org/acgmeweb/Portals/0/PFAssets/ProgramResources/480-Urology-Case-Log-Info_.pdf. Accessed April 15, 2015.

medical field that combines conservative and surgical techniques and involves diagnostics reaching from ultrasonography to bacteriology to very differentiated and complex surgical interventions.

3.17 Gynecology and Obstetrics

Just as in most other areas, gynecologic diagnostics begins with close examination. For example, in dermatology, young and old patients, men and women, can be examined at any time. However, the gynecologic examination is a physical examination of the female genital area and must be performed with sensitivity and compassion (**Fig. 3.25**). The examination typically includes a physical examination of the patient, histories of the patient and her family, her gynecologic history, including her menstrual cycle and possible deviations, and an examination of the breasts. Breast cancer screening has become a standard procedure in most Western countries. Establishment of this procedure is justified: thanks to breast cancer screening, many women with breast cancer have been identified early enough that timely treatment and breast-conserving surgery were possible.

In many countries, including the United States, breast cancer treatment is part of oncology, and breast surgery is part of plastic surgery. In the West, breast cancer is the most common type of cancer among females. In a growing number of specialized clinics, gynecologists focus on diseases of the breast, particularly breast cancer. Comparable to other areas, it has been shown that those physicians who perform many surgeries in one particular area are postoperatively more successful than physicians who cover the broad range of the entire field. Breast cancer diagnostics and therapy have become multimodal. In diagnostics, an experienced radiologist should be consulted who can recognize changes in breast tissue. We learn during pathology that breasts change in the course of a woman's life. They grow during puberty, are subject to hormonal fluctuations, and are important glands during lactation periods. Organs subject to change, build-up, and restructuring, as well as growing and shrinking, are more prone to tumoral degeneration than other tissues. This statement should not be overgeneralized but is aimed at helping the medical student understand the nature of breast cancer. Genetics and genetic markers are responsible for 5% of breast cancer and should be tested in cases of known disposition. Integral parts of treat-

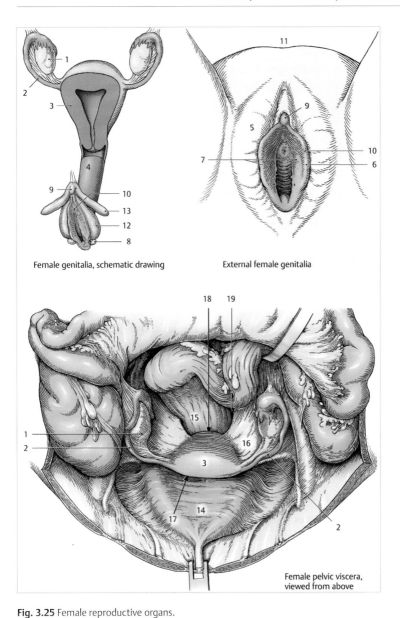

Female genitalia, schematic drawing

External female genitalia

Female pelvic viscera,
viewed from above

Fig. 3.25 Female reproductive organs.
1 Ovary, 2 Uterine tube, 3 Uterus, 4 Vagina, 5 Labium majus, 6 Labium minus, 7
Vestibule of vagina, 8 Vestibular glands, 9 Clitoris, 10 Urethral orifice, 11 Mons
pubis, 12 Bulb of vestibule, 13 Crus of clitoris, 14 Urinary bladder, 15 Rectum, 16
Broad ligament of the uterus, 17 Vesicouterine pouch, 18 Rectouterine pouch (pouch
of Douglas), 19 Rectouterine fold

ment include nuclear medicine for identification of the sentinel lymph node, radiation therapy, oncology, and psycho-oncology. Breast cancer diagnostics is an example of neccessary multidisciplinary involvement in diagnostics and therapy. This includes postoperative rehabilitation. Women must learn how to live with this disease. For example, they must be provided with counseling following a total or partial mastectomy. The integration of psychosocial aspects is crucial to the course of the disease and healing process.

The physician certainly remembers the anatomic and topographic introduction to the location and relation of gynecologic structures, including the uterus, vagina, vulva, bladder, and the adnexa as well as the fallopian tubes and ovaries. These structures form another area of gynecologic diagnostics and therapy.

Uterine diseases include congenital anomalies and anomalies of presentation. Inflammations and endometriosis, which is the growth of the uterine mucosa outside of the uterus, are common disorders. The most frequent uterine tumors are cervical and endometrial cancers. Etiologically speaking, estrogen is a decisive factor in endometrial cancer, whereas human papillomavirus (HPV) plays a role in cervical cancer. The vagina and vulva can present with anomalies such as atresia or hyperplasia. Some of the most frequently seen disorders in this area include vulvitis, colitis, and vaginal and vulvar tumors. Human papillomavirus–induced vulvar tumors are increasing in incidence. In particular, the adnexa of the uterus and the ovaries may be affected by ovarian cysts, tumors, or ovarian cancer.

In 1847, the Hungarian gynecologist Ignaz Semmelweis discovered the cause of childbed (puerperal) fever. It is not an internal disease, but rather germs were transmitted on the hands of physicians and nurses to the women. Physicians at that time did not accept this explanation of the cause of childbed fever, so Semmelweis was initially ignored (see Semmelweis 1861). This should be an example for subsequent generations of physicians to hold on to their convictions if something is in the best interest of the patient, even if the consequences are frustrating. At times we must fight for a treatment, a general change, or an individual change in therapy. Usually, success proves us right.

Let us recall Hippocrates from Kos, particularly the fourth paragraph of the Hippocratic Oath: "I will not give a lethal drug to anyone if I am asked, nor will I advise such a plan; and similarly I will not give a woman a pessary to cause an abortion." For more than 2,000 years, this ethical attitude has remained widely exemplary for physicians.

Semmelweis's finding is still relevant today! Still in modern times, premature infants are treated in intensive care units contaminated with pathogens. They become infected and die in the modern clinics of the Western world. Medicine changes and medical research and development are in a constant state of progress, but fundamentals stand the test of time.

While most medical specialty areas are divided into subspecialties, gynecology and obstetrics are still a combined specialty. However, there are tendencies to separate these areas and some large clinics have done so. Obstetrics is a gratifying medical specialty. No one will ever forget the moments in the delivery room witnessing the birth of a child. A regular birth is as normal and uncomplicated as life itself. Difficulties arise with irregularities during the pregnancy, placental anomalies, or in the event of multiple pregnancies. In particular, premature placental separation and premature water breaking are challenges for the obstetrician.

Due to the possible complications in gynecology, certain knowledge is of particular importance, such as coagulation disorders, blood transfusions, and blood typing. The attendance of approximately 500 unsupervised deliveries is recommended for the sound education of a physician in postgraduate gynecological training. Knowledge of gynecologic endocrinology, particularly infertility counseling as it relates to family counseling, is an integral element of gynecologic training.

The field of obstetrics/gynecology combines different aspects of diagnosis and therapy, including the challenges of childbirth, manual challenges during surgery, menstrual symptoms, issues during pregnancy, and, at times, cancer therapy.

3.18 Ophthalmology

Ophthalmology is a small and limited specialty. The physician must combine manual and intellectual abilities. Patients identify their well-being with good vision, and many consider impaired vision to be a more serious condition than other physical ailments. In anatomy and physiology, the student learned about eyes and vision. More than in any other field, expertise in this medical specialty is focused on the anatomic structures of its subject. It is crucial to understand and describe the vascular supply of the eye, its position in the skull, and its surrounding structures. Six of the 12 cranial nerves are connected to the eyes. No other medical specialty revolves around the skull and its individual bones to this extent. The most significant square millimeters in the body make up the fovea centralis in the retina; it is the area of the eye with the highest sensitivity to fine detail. In the center of the retina is the optic nerve, which contains the ganglion cell axons running to the brain, and incoming blood vessels that open into the retina (**Fig. 3.26**).

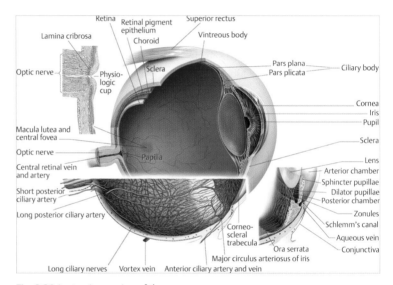

Fig. 3.26 Anatomic overview of the eye.

Ophthalmology is a medical field in which diagnosis and later therapy are performed under the microscope. In ophthalmology, the patient immediately recognizes surgical success, such as the implantation of an artificial lens. Surgical alterations to the cornea are instantly obvious to patients and colleagues who can then judge the quality of the surgery. Common ophthalmologic diseases include diseases of the eyelids, tear ducts, and conjunctiva. In this field, the physician frequently encounters bacterial and viral infections, including trachoma, which is common in the tropics. Globally, corneal diseases are among the most frequent causes of vision loss. In addition to congenital diseases, infections frequently cause corneal changes, which can also lead to blindness. In Western countries, cataracts are another common cause of vision loss. Increase in life expectancy comes with an increase of degenerative processes in tendons and ligaments, but also in other tissues such as the lens. The clouding of the lens in various areas is often irreversible. Modern optic surgery allows for the implantation of new lenses in outpatient clinics. The artificial lens comes with tiny hooks. After the clouded part of the lens is removed via phacoemulsification, the new lens is implanted into the remaining capsular bag. This intervention has spared many patients from losing their vision. However, currently, the cornea cannot be replaced by an artificial implantation but only by another human cornea. Today, an artificial replacement is still not possible.

Most ophthalmologists in private practice do not perform surgeries. Ophthalmologic surgeries are typically limited to ophthalmology departments of hospitals. Ophthalmologic interventions are usually performed under the microscope and require a high tolerance threshold, absolute concentration, and precision dexterity from the surgeon. Students wishing to enter the field may be required to perform surgical exercises under the microscope on the eyes of animals such as rats and pigs. Physicians who enjoy performing surgery and are capable of clamping an aorta, cutting it, and suturing it again under the microscope may find their calling in ophthalmology.

The increasing incidence of diabetes mellitus, a widespread disease in the West, is typically accompanied by an increased incidence of retinal circulatory disorders. In diabetes, the delicate vessels of the retina are eventually destroyed along with their blood supply. These vessels represent one of the most sensitive structures in the human body, and their destruction results in degeneration of the retina. In most cases, this proliferating process cannot be halted. Similar to the cornea, there are very few options for compensation.

Glaucoma is also increasing in incidence. Acute glaucoma is one of the very few emergencies in ophthalmology. It must be immediately treated with acetazolamide/pilocarpine.

Every ophthalmologist must possess the armamentarium of knowledge relating to internal medicine. Apart from the knowledge regarding bacterial and viral pathogens, essential activities of an ophthalmologist include therapy for eye problems related to hypertension-related diseases, rheumatoid disorders, and diabetes mellitus.

Ophthalmology offers diverse activities and interfaces to the fields of the physiology, anatomy, neurology, bacteriology, and neurosurgery. Every ophthalmologist and every family physician must be able to perform ophthalmoscopy. Sometimes an ophthalmologist must consult on matters of fraud. Some years ago, there was the case of a 60-year-old patient who collected early retirement for years due to vision loss caused by an accident. When his pension insurance caseworker retired and a new caseworker was assigned, the new caseworker became concerned when he noticed that the man acted as a referee at soccer games every weekend. He was highly valued as a referee because he noticed every little detail on the field. Thus, an ophthalmologist was consulted and helped to prove the fraud.

In Western countries, the respective medical boards and examination offices include differing interventions in their catalogs of surgical procedures. In Germany, for example, this catalog requires the following surgical procedures: 100 local and regional anesthesias; 50 surgeries to eyelids and tear ducts, particularly correction of entropion and ectropion, eyelid muscle surgery, and stretching and stricture excision of tear ducts; 50 surgeries on conjunctiva and cornea, particularly removal of foreign bodies and sutures; 25 simple intraocular interventions, particularly paracentesis, iridectomy, cryo- and laser cycloablation, and cryoretinopexy; 10 interventions to the rectal eye muscles; 50 laser surgeries to the anterior segment of the eye; 100 laser surgeries to the retina and surgical assistance in intraocular interventions, including retinal and vascular surgeries, eye muscle surgeries of higher difficulty levels such as cataract, glaucoma, retinal detachment surgeries, vitrectomy, enucleation, keratoplasty; and plastic reconstructive interventions on at least 100 patients. In the United States, residents are required to achieve the number of procedures determined by the ACGME.

Ophthalmology may be the right fit for someone with surgical dexterity who is in search of a highly specialized field, who can concentrate on a few millimeters over extended periods of time, and wants to treat old and young patients alike.

3.19 Otolaryngology

Otolaryngology (also referred to as otorhinolaryngology) is a specialty predominantly defined by anatomic structures and physiologic functions. Therefore, a thorough knowledge of anatomy and the topography of muscles, bones, and vessels as well as the nerves of the neck, face, and skull are essential. Physiology occupies a large part of diagnostics in otolaryngology. Physiologic processes such as hearing high- and low-pitched tones and the mechanical transmission of acoustic waves via the eardrum and middle ear to the electrical stimulation of the cochlea, swallowing processes, organs of speech formation, as well as the ability to taste and smell, must be understood. Conductive hearing disorders must be differentiated from perceptive hearing disorders by conducting varying types of tests. The same applies to symptoms of central or vestibular vertigo. Vertigo that originates in the central nervous system produces symptoms such as blacking out, nausea, and drowsiness. Vestibular vertigo is usually perceived as rotary vertigo. With the aid of a scope, every physician should be able to examine the larynx. In thyroid surgery, students were introduced to the sensory and motor supplies through the superior laryngeal nerve and the recurrent laryngeal nerve. We also know that injuries to the recurrent laryngeal nerve can cause vocal cord paralysis and that, in cases of bilateral paralysis, tracheotomy alone may save the patient from suffocating.

We can tell that, once again, anatomy and physiology are the foundation for comprehending functions and subsequent diseases (due to malfunction) in the field of otolaryngology. Otolaryngology is an interface between pathology, pharmacology, oncology, radiology, neurology, neurosurgery, and pediatrics. For example, children may commonly present with otolaryngeal infections (the most frequent infection during childhood is otitis media).

Emergencies include bleeding and shortness of breath in the area of the throat due to trauma, foreign bodies, or infections with subsequent swelling that constricts the air passages. Otolaryngology is the leading medical specialty for dramatic and life-threatening emergencies in children. Children try to (and do) put everything in their mouths, which can lead to foreign body aspiration and dangerous respiratory distress. A thorough and swift evaluation of the situation and immediate removal of the foreign body are often life-saving maneuvers. Particularly among infants, bacterial epiglottitis can become life-threatening. We must differentiate between epiglottitis and pseudocroup. Swelling of the subglottic space caused by a viral infection can also become acutely life-threatening during the first four years of life. In these cases, it is necessary to keep calm. As a result of the increased incidence of allergies, which are often cased by environmental factors, cases of allergic edema in the mouth and throat cavity are on the rise. Patients with allergic edema also require thorough evaluation and determined action by the physician.

The work of the otolaryngologist requires a sensitive approach to pediatric diseases and compassion regarding the situation of older patients with degenerative diseases, dementia, or hearing loss. Few other medical specialties offer the same range of diagnostics and therapeutic methods as otolaryngology. There is great variety in differentiated otolaryngeal diagnostics. Clinical examination, ultrasonography, and endoscopy are essential. Diagnostics such as conventional X-ray diagnostic, CT, and MRI are vital for detecting and identifying the presence of a tumor and its dimensions. Additional procedures include audiologic diagnostics, such as tuning-fork tests, threshold and speech audiograms, impedance measurement, otoacoustic emissions, and electrical response audiometry. The broad range of diagnostics includes very diverse approaches such as electrical procedures for the various types of cranial nerve examinations (**Fig. 3.27**), ventilation testing in shortness of breath, and stroboscopic analysis of the vibrations of the vocal folds, just to name a few.

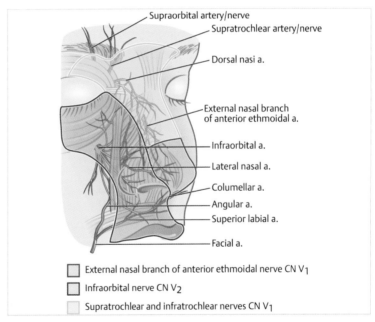

Supraorbital artery/nerve
Supratrochlear artery/nerve
Dorsal nasi a.
External nasal branch of anterior ethmoidal a.
Infraorbital a.
Lateral nasal a.
Columellar a.
Angular a.
Superior labial a.
Facial a.

☐ External nasal branch of anterior ethmoidal nerve CN V_1
☐ Infraorbital nerve CN V_2
☐ Supratrochlear and infratrochlear nerves CN V_1

Fig. 3.27 Schematic drawing demonstrating the blood supply and innervation of the external nose.

In diseases of the mouth and throat area, the otolaryngologist works closely with an oral and maxillofacial surgeon. When presented with mucosal changes, the otolaryngologist must recognize leukoplakia as a possible pretumorous condition. Oropharyngeal inflammations, acute pharyngitis, and tonsillitis must be closely observed. Streptococci spread can lead to secondary diseases. Sometimes tonsillectomy is the only therapeutic alternative to antibiotic treatment. Nicotine and alcohol abuse increase the incidence of tumors in the oropharyngeal area.

Just like in other medical specialties, major otolaryngeal tumor surgeries should be and are exclusively performed in specialized clinics. Surgeries for cancer of the pharynx or larynx should be carried out in well-established otolaryngology departments by experienced surgeons. Multidisciplinary collaboration is essential and includes the staff from the oncology, radiology, oral and maxillofacial surgery, and neurosurgery departments. Pharyngeal and laryngeal tumors frequently require very involved and invasive interventions, a fact that becomes obvious when considering that all of the nerves and vessels in the body travel through the neck to the trunk. Surgeries in the neck area require particular sensitivity. Extirpation of lymph nodes has been a subject of debate because it is a rather disfiguring surgery. Thus, close collaboration with other medical disciplines is vital in the field of otolaryngology.

Inflammation of the nose (rhinitis) may have a variety of etiologic causes, including simple acute viral rhinitis, lupus erythematosus, leprosy, or inflammations caused by tropical diseases. Sinusitis can be highly encumbering for patients. Psychological guidance is an important aspect of the healing process.

Diseases of the external ear are frequently found in boxers and wrestlers. They manifest as swollen and chondroitic changes, also called cauliflower ear. Ear diagnostics and therapy include conditions like basal cell carcinoma and melanoma, trauma to the middle ear, and various forms of otitis media. In all types of diagnostics and therapy in the close vicinity of nerves, the facial nerve must be considered. Frequent causes of vertigo are vestibular disorders such as Meniere's disease, which is a triad of rotary vertigo, unilateral tinnitus, and unilateral hearing loss due to hydrops of the internal layer of the labyrinth. Sudden deafness is a unilateral sudden loss of hearing. It may occur in conjunction with allergies or viral infections. Listening to loud music with headphones has caused below average hearing capacity in many young people. Here, too, the otolaryngologist should step in preventively.

Phoniatrics and pediatric audiology have developed as subspecialties of otolaryngology addressing dysphonia and speech disorders; thus, collaboration with psychosomatic medicine specialists and child and adolescent psychiatrists is necessary. The subspecialty includes exact diagnostics of motor function, language and speech exercises, discerning of perceptual disorders in children, and voice therapy, which is the teaching of proper articulation.

Otolaryngology is an interesting and sophisticated specialty. It covers the entire medical range from inflammations to tumors in the young and old, and it may be practiced in private practice or in a clinic. This field comes with many prerequisites for a gratifying career.

3.20 Forensic Pathology

Forensic pathologists work at the interface of medicine and law. Their tasks can include determining the cause, manner (including whether the death was from natural, unnatural, or undetermined causes), and time of death. Particularly challenging cases for determining time of death sometimes involve a decedent whose body has begun to display significant decay prior to being found by the proper authorities. The information gleaned from the case may be presented in court as medical opinion for legal reasons, matters of public record, or for other purposes beyond the scope of this book.

Every physician should be able to conduct an autopsy. There are three reliable signs of death: livor mortis, rigor mortis, and putrefaction. Every physician must recognize these three reliable signs of death. Patients whose dying process was accompanied by medical care and who died of a natural cause do not require an autopsy. Forensic autopsy should generally be performed on unidentified decedents, when discovering decedents, or following the death of a patient in the emergency department. Clinical autopsy may clarify the cause of death and serves the purpose of ascertaining the diagnosis and revealing possible crimes. If consent is provided, an autopsy should be ordered if there is any doubt about the cause and manner of death in a patient.

The autopsy and the death certificate are also part of confirming death when someone dies in a long-term care facility. Collaboration between long-term care facility staff and the physician issuing the death certificate must be discriminating and judicial. Case in point, in 2010 a very well-liked, friendly, and thoughtful caretaker in a German long-term care facility committed a series of murders. In one of the deaths, a physician improperly conducted the autopsy while the decedent was still dressed! As a rule in Germany, autopsy must be conducted on the naked corpse in a well-lit location. When this caretaker called on the physician once again on a Saturday morning so that the physician would issue a death certificate, the physician declined due to a cold and sent a colleague. The colleague arrived in the afternoon to finish the autopsy. The caretaker was quite irritated. The replacement physician insisted that the decedent be undressed in order to perform the autopsy. This was when he noticed that the decedent had two new puncture sites at the medial cubital vein. At this point, he discontinued his examination and ordered a forensic autopsy, where it was determined that the cause of death was an air embolism and the manner of death was the injection of air into the right cubital vein. During the ensuing criminal investigation, investigators noticed that 20 patients had died, predominantly women, over the last 1.5 years. Times of death were compared to the working schedule of the caretaker and a correlation was immediately detected, and the caretaker was convicted of murder. This case serves to illustrate the importance of proper autopsy methods and the type of forensic challenges that may result from improperly conducting medical procedures.

The fascinating field of poisoning also belongs to forensic pathology. We were introduced to poisonings in pharmacology. We keep meeting them in crime stories, but, in reality, the number of poisoners has drastically declined. Instead, alcohol and illicit drug intoxications are on the rise. Consuming alcohol and safely driving a vehicle are mutually exclusive. However, many fatal motor vehicle collisions are related to alcohol use. There are still startling numbers of people who abuse heroin, cocaine, and methamphetamines. Therapeutic intervention in cases of heroin addiction is possible through the administration of methadone, buprenorphine, and naloxone. In most cases, drug intoxication must be symptomatically treated. The frequent incidences of poisoning with sleeping pills are declining because those currently available on the market have a wide margin of safety. Infrequently occurring poisoning with arsenic, gold, or mercury is treated with British anti-Lewisite (BAL). Copper, cobalt, zinc, or lead poisonings are treated with various forms of chelation therapy, for example, with ethylenediaminetetraacetic acid (EDTA). Organophosphate poisonings are traditionally treated with atropine, sometimes in combination with low-dose pralidoxime. Fortunately, the declining numbers of cyanide poisonings are treated with intravenous hydroxocobalamin and sodium thiosulfate and sodium nitrite.

Forensic pathology can include responding to coroner inquests into blunt or sharp force injuries, suffocation, gunshot wounds, deaths as a result of heat or cold, as well as child abuse and infanticide, medical/actuarial science, and biologic trace analysis (e.g., blood, sperm, and vaginal secretions). With the aid of DNA technology, by comparing DNA findings on victims or crime scenes with DNA of suspects, matches can be found and offenders convicted. This is particularly helpful in murder or child abuse cases. Sexual perversion, which we learned about in psychiatry, also belongs to forensic pathology. Usually in terms of medical opinion, the involvement of a forensic pathologist is required in cases of sexual assault, sexual perversions, voyeurism, sadomasochism, and the sexual or mental abuse of minors.

Physicians who do not miss medical consultation and who do not mind having to perform hours of autopsy are a good fit for forensic pathology. In their work, forensic pathologists focus on answering questions that may have gone unanswered, providing closure to loved ones, and solving crime. Most forensic pathologists work at universities, governmental institutions, or as medical examiners.

Section III
Appendix

Bibliography

If you want to test a man's character,
give him power.

Abraham Lincoln

Accreditation Council for Graduate Medical Education (ACGME) website. Available at: http://www.acgme.org. Accessed April 15, 2015

Ackerknecht EH. A Short History of Medicine. New York, NY: Thieme Publishers; 1967

Addison T. On the Constitutional and Local Effects of Disease of the Suprarenal Capsules. London: Samuel Highley; 1855

Adler A. The Practice and Theory of Individual Psychology. Radin P, trans. London: Routledge; 1925

Agency of Healthcare Research and Quality (AHRQ) (USA). Healthcare Cost and Utilization Project. Available at: http://hcupnet.ahrq.gov/. Accessed April 15, 2015

American Lung Association. State of Lung Disease in Diverse Communities 2010. Available at: http://www.lung.org/assets/documents/publications/lung-disease-data/solddc_2010.pdf. Accessed April 15, 2015

Andress C. Rudolf Virchow. Leben und Ethos eines großen Arztes. Munich: Langen Müller; 2002

Barnard C. One Life. Munich: Scherz; 1969

Birkmeyer J, Siewers AE, Finlaysun EVA, et al. Hospital volume and surgical mortality in the United States. N Engl J Med. 2002;346(15):1128–1137

Bleuler PE. Dementia praecox oder Gruppe der Schizophrenien. In: Aschaffenburg G (ed.). Handbuch der Psychiatrie. Leipzig/Vienna: F. Deuticke; 1911

Bleuler PE. Lehrbuch der Psychiatrie. Berlin: Springer; 1983

Bliss M. Harvey Cushing. A Life in Surgery. Oxford/New York, NY: Oxford University Press; 2005

Brunicardi SC, Andersen DK. Principals of Surgery. 8th ed. New York, NY: McGraw-Hill Medical Publishing Division; 2005

Christian PE, Waterstram-Rich KM. Nuclear Medicine and PET/CT: Technology and Techniques. 7th ed. London: Mosby; 2011

Cushing HW. From a Surgeon's Journal 1915–1918. Boston, MA: Little, Brown, and Company; 1936

Cushing HW. A Visit to Le Puy-en-Velay. An Illustrated Diary. Cleveland, OH: The Rowfant Club; 1944

DESTATIS 2013. Fallpauschalenbezogene Krankenhausstatistik (DRG-Statistik). Operationen und Prozeduren der vollstationären Patientinnen und Patienten in Krankenhäusern. Statistisches Bundesamt, Wiesbaden 2014.

di Maio V. Forensic Pathology. 2nd ed. Boca Raton, FL/London: CRC Press; 2001

Dorland. Dorland's Illustrated Medical Dictionary. 31st ed. Philadelphia, PA: Saunders; 2007

Dussault G, Fronteira I, Cabral J. Migration of Health Personnel in the WHO European Region. Copenhagen: WHO Regional Office for Europe; 2009. Available at: http://www.euro.who.int/en/health-topics/Health-systems/health-workforce/publications2/2009/migration-of-health-personnel-in-the-who-european-region-2009. Accessed November 10, 2014.

Feix J, ed. Herodot. Historien. Düsseldorf: Artemis & Winkler; 2004

Foucault M. Madness and Civilization: A History of Insanity in the Age of Reason. Howard R, trans. New York, NY: Pantheon Books; 1965

Frankl VE. Collected Works. Batthyany A, Biller K, Fizzotti E, eds. Vienna: Böhlau; 2005

Frenk J, Chen L, Bhutta ZA, et al. Health professionals for a new century. Transforming education to strengthen health systems in an interdependent world. Lancet. 2010;376:1923–1958

Frohlich E. Rypins' Medical Licensure Examinations. Philadelphia, PA: J.B. Lippincott Co.; 1985

Gebhardt U. Sichere Pille für kleine Patienten. Neue Züricher Zeitung. October 10, 2010

Geisler LS. Arzt und Patient—Begegnung im Gespräch. 4th ed. Frankfurt/Main: Pharma; 2002

Global Health Workforce Alliance (GHWA)/World Health Organization (WHO). A Universal Truth: No Health Without a Workforce. Third Global Forum on Human Resources for Health Report. Geneva: World Health Organization; 2014. Available at: http://www.who.int/work-

forcealliance/knowledge/resources/hrhreport2013/en/.   Accessed
November 10, 2014.

Goschler C. Rudolf Virchow. Mediziner-Antropologe-Politiker. Cologne,
Weimar, Vienna: Böhlau; 2009

Graafland M, Schraagen JM, Schijven MP. Systematic review of serious
games for medical education and surgical skills training. Br J Surg.
2012;99:1322–1330

Graves RJ. New observed affection of the thyroid gland in females. Lond
Med Surg J. 1835;7:516–517

Guilford JP. Cognitive psychology's ambiguities: Some suggested rem-
edies. Psychol Rev. 1982;89(1):48–59

Harvey W. Exercitatio Anatomica de Motu Cordis et Sanguinis in Animalibus. Frankfurt/Main: Wilhelm Fitzer; 1628

Haustein KO. Tobacco or Health. Berlin: Springer; 2003

Holmes TH, Rahe RH. The social readjustment rating scale. J Psychosom
Res. 1967;11(2):213–218

International Agency for Research on Cancer/World Health Organization. Globocan 2012: Estimated Cancer Incidence, Mortality and
Prevalence Worldwide in 2012/Prediction. Available at: http://globo-
can.iarc.fr/Pages/burden_sel.aspx. Accessed November 10, 2014

Jaspers K. Die Idee des Arztes. Munich: Piper; 1958

Jaspers K. Die Idee der Universität. Berlin: Springer; 1961

Jellinek EM. The Disease Concept of Alcoholism. New Haven, CT: Mill-
house Press; 1960

Kaiser LR, Singhal S. Essentials of Thoracic Surgery. Philadelphia, PA:
Elsevier-Mosby; 2007

Kant E. Critique of Pure Reason. Cambridge, UK: Cambridge University
Press; 1999

Kennedy JF. To Turn to Die. New York, NY: Harper & Brothers; 1962

Kerres M. Mediendidaktik: Konzeption und Entwicklung medienge-
stützter Lernangebote. 3rd new ed. Munich: Oldenbourg; 2012

Keys TE. The History of Surgery and Anesthesia. New York, NY: Dover
Publications; 1945

Kneucker AW. Richtlinien einer Philosophie der Medizin. Vienna: Wilhelm Maudrich 1949

Knoop KJ, Stack LB. Storrow AB. Atlas of Emergency Medicine. New York,
NY: McGraw-Hill Medical Publishing Division; 2005

Koch R. Die Aetiologie der Milzbrand-Krankheit, begründet auf die Entwicklungsgeschichte des Bacillus anthracis. Beitr Biol Pflanzen. 1876;2:277–310

Koch R. Die Aetiologie der Tuberkulose. Berliner Klinischen Wochenschrift No. 15. 1882:221–30

Koch R. Die Aetiologie der Tuberkulose. Mittheilungen aus dem Kaiserlichen Gesundheitsamte, Vol. 2. Berlin: Norddeutsche Buchdruckerei und Verlagsanstalt; 1884:1–88

Kolb DA. Experiental Learning: Experience as the Source of Learning and Development. Englewood Cliffs, NJ: Prentice-Hall, Inc.; 1984

Krukemeyer MG. Kultur der Medizin. Spuren, Wege und Ziele. Stuttgart: Schattauer; 2011

Krukemeyer MG, Lison AE, eds. Transplantationsmedizin. Berlin: de Gruyter; 2006

Krukemeyer MG, Moellenhoff G, eds. Endoprothetik. 3rd ed. Berlin: de Gruyter; 2012

Krukemeyer MG, Pueschel K. Leichenschau und Todesbescheinigung. Ein Vademekum für die Rechtssicherheit des Arztes. Med Welt 2005;6:270-277

Krukemeyer MG, Spiegel HU, eds. Chirurgische Forschung. Stuttgart: Thieme 2005

Kuebler-Ross E. On Death and Dying. New York, NY: The Macmillan Company 1969

Leriche R. Philosophie der Chirurgie. Zurich: Rascher; 1954

Loscalzo J, Jameson JL, Hauser SL, et al. Harrison's Principles of Internal Medicine. 18th ed. New York, NY: McGraw-Hill; 2011

Maddrey EC, Sorrell MS. Transplantation of the Liver. Norwalk, CT: Appleton and Lange; 1995

Mathers CD, Loncar D. Projections of global mortality and burden of disease from 2002 to 2030. PLoS Med. 2006;3(11):e422

McMoran Wilson C. Winston Churchill — The Struggle for Survival 1940–1965. London: Constable; 1966

Meerwein F. Das ärztliche Gespräch. Bern: Hans Huber; 1969

Milgram S. Obedience to Authority. New York, NY: Harper & Row; 1974

Mirzayan R. Itamura JM. Trauma of Shoulder and Elbow. New York, NY: Thieme Publishers; 2004

Munthe A. The Story of San Michele. Berlin: Ullstein; 1991

OECD. OECD Factbook 2011–2012: Economic, Environmental and Social Statistics. Paris: OECD Publishing; 2011. Available at: http://www.oecd-ilibrary.org/economics/oecd-factbook-2011-2012_factbook-2011-en. Accessed November 10, 2014

OECD. Health at a Glance 2013: OECD Indicators. Paris: OECD Publishing; 2013. Available at: http://www.oecd-ilibrary.org/social-issues-migration-health/health-at-a-glance-2013_health_glance-2013-en. Accessed November 10, 2014

OECD. OECD Factbook 2014: Economic, Environmental and Social Statistics. Paris: OECD Publishing; 2014. Available at: http://www.oecd-ilibrary.org/economics/oecd-factbook_18147364. Accessed November 10, 2014

OECD. Statistics website. Available at: http://stats.oecd.org. Accessed November 10, 2014

Paracelsus. Septem Defensiones. Die Selbstverteidigung eines Außenseiters. Poerksen G., trans. Basel: Schwabe; 2003

Penzoldt F. Lehrbuch der klinischen Arzneibehandlung: für Studierende und Ärzte. 8th ed. Jena: Fischer; 1915

Penzoldt F. Ärztliche Visite. In: Hansen K, ed. Lesebuch für Ärzte. Berlin: Karl H. Henssel Verlag; 1950

Peters W, Pasvol G. Tropical Medicine and Parasitology. 5th ed. London: Mosby; 2002

Pickup RW, Saunders JR. Molecular approaches to environmental microbiology. London: Ellis Horwood; 1996

Ringel E. Die subjektive Wirklichkeit des Patienten. Vienna: Facultas; 1982

Ringel E. Selbstschädigung durch Neurose. Vienna: Herder; 1983

Roe M, ed. Speeches and Letters by Abraham Lincoln. London: J.M. Dent; 1949

Roentgen WC. Ueber eine neue Art von Strahlen [On a new kind of rays]. Vorläufige Mittheilung. Aus den Sitzungsberichten der Würzburger Physik.-medic. Gesellschaft. Würzburg: Stahel'sche K. Hof- und Universitätsbuch- und Kunsthandlung; 1895:137–147

Russell B. A History of Western Philosophy. London: Allen & Unwin; 1950

Sauerbruch F. Das war mein Leben. München: Droemer Knaur; 1995

Schadewaldt H. Arzt und Patient in antiker und frühchristlicher Sicht. Med Klein. 1964;59:146–152

Schaefer C. Modelle einer erfolgreichen Implementierung elektronischer und anderer Lernmaterialien in die Lehre. In: Krukemeyer MG, ed. Aus- und Weiterbildung in der klinischen Medizin. Didaktik und Ausbildungskonzepte. Stuttgart: Schattauer; 2012

Schaefer H. Plädoyer für eine neue Medizin. Munich: Piper; 1979

Schettler FG. Lehrbuch der Inneren Medizin. Stuttgart: Thieme Publishers; 1985

Schippergers H. Rudolf Virchow. Hamburg: Rowohlt; 1994

Schweitzer A. Gesammelte Werke in fünf Bänden. Grabs R, ed. Munich: Beck; 1974

Semmelweis IP. Die Aetiologie, der Begriff und die Prophylaxe des Kindbettfiebers. Pest/Vienna/Leipzig: Hartleben; 1861

Sherlock S, Summerfield JA. A Colour Atlas of Liver Disease. 2nd ed. London: Wolfe Publishing; 1991

Siyam A, Dal Poz MR, eds. Migration of Health Workers: The WHO Code of Practice and the Global Economic Crisis. Geneva: World Health Organization; 2014. Available at: http://www.who.int/hrh/migration/migration_book/en/. Accessed November 11, 2014.

Siyam A, Dal Poz MR, eds. Migration of Health Workers: The WHO Code of Practice and the Global Economic Crisis. Geneva: World Health Organization; 2014

Souba WW, Wilmore DD. Surgical Research. San Diego, CA: Academic Press; 2001

Thomson EH. Harvey Cushing. Surgeon, Author, Artist. New York, NY: Henry Schuman; 1950

Tjadens F, Weilandt C, Eckert J, et al. Mobility of Health Professionals. Health Systems, Work Conditions, Patterns of Health Workers' Mobility and Implications for Policy Makers. Bonn: WIAD (Scientific Institute of the Medical Association of German Doctors); 2012

Townsend CM. Beauchamp RD, Evers BM, et al. Textbook of Surgery: The Biological Basis of Modern Surgical Practice. 19th ed. Philadelphia, PA: Saunders; 2012

Troidel H, McKneally MF, Molder ES, et al. Surgical Research. 3rd ed. Heidelberg: Springer; 1987

Uflacker R. Atlas of Vascular Anatomy. Philadelphia, PA: Williams and Wilkins; 1997

UNAIDS. The Gap Report. Geneva: United Nations; 2014. Available at: http://www.unaids.org/sites/default/files/media_asset/UNAIDS_Gap_report_en.pdf. Accessed April 9, 2015

United Nations Office on Drugs and Crime. World Drug Report 2014 (United Nations Publication, Sales No. E.14.XI.7), © United Nations, June 2014. Vienna: ONODC; 2014:1–6. Available at: http://www.unodc.org/wdr2014/. Accessed November 10, 2014.

Vasold M. Rudolf Virchow. Der große Arzt und Politiker. Frankfurt: Fischer; 1990

Vesalius A. De Humani Corporis Fabrica. Basel: Johannes Oporinus; 1543

Virchow R. Die Cellularpathologie in ihrer Begründung auf physiologische und pathologische Gewebelehre. 3rd ed. Berlin: Hirschwald; 1862

von Basedow CA. Exophthalmus durch Hypertrophie des Zellgewebes in der Augenhöhle. Wochenschrift für die gesammte Heilkunde; 1840:13–14, 197–204, 220–228

Wachsmuth W. Leben mit dem Jahrhundert. Berlin: Springer; 1985

Weill FS, Manco-Johnson ML. Imaging of Abdominal and Pelvic Anatomy. New York, NY: Churchill Livingstone; 1997

Wesiack W, ed. Entwicklungstendenzen in der psychosomatischen Medizin. Eine Ringvorlesung. Professor Doktor Thure von Uexküll zu seinem 80. Geburtstag. Berlin, Heidelberg, New York, London, Paris, Tokyo: Springer; 1988

WHO. Preamble to the Constitution of the World Health Organization; 1946. Available at: http://www.who.int/governance/eb/who_constitution_en.pdf. Accessed April 15, 2015

WHO. The Global Burden of Disease: 2004 Update. Geneva: World Health Organization; 2004. Available at: http://www.who.int/healthinfo/global_burden_disease/2004_report_update/en/. Accessed April 15, 2015

WHO. The World Health Report 2006: Working Together for Health. Geneva: World Health Organization; 2006. Available at: http://www.who.int/whr/2006/en/. Accessed 10 November, 2014

WHO. Transformative Scale up of Health Professional Education. An Effort to Increase the Numbers of Health Professionals and to Strengthen Their Impact on Population Health. Geneva: World Health Organization; 2011. Available at: http://whqlibdoc.who.int/hq/2011/WHO_HSS_HRH_HEP2011.01_eng.pdf. November 31, 2014

WHO. Global Report: Mortality Attributable to Tobacco. Geneva: World Health Organization; 2012. Available at: http://www.who.int/tobacco/publications/surveillance/rep_mortality_attibutable/en/. Accessed 10 November 2014

WHO. Cardiovascular diseases (CVDs). Fact sheet no. 317. Geneva: World Health Organization; 2013. Available at: http://www.who.int/mediacentre/factsheets/fs317/en/. Accessed November 10, 2014

WHO. Chronic obstructive pulmonary disease (COPD). Fact sheet no. 315. Geneva: World Health Organization; 2013. Available at: http://www.who.int/mediacentre/factsheets/fs315/en/. Accessed 10 November, 2014

WHO. Diarrhoeal disease. Fact sheet no. 330. Geneva: World Health Organization; 2013. Available at: http://www.who.int/mediacentre/factsheets/fs330/en. Accessed November 10, 2014

WHO. Global Tuberculosis Report 2013. Geneva: World Health Organization; 2013. Available at: http://www.who.int/tb/publications/global_report/en. Accessed November 10, 2014

WHO. World Malaria Report: 2013. Geneva: World Health Organization; 2013. Available at http://www.who.int/malaria/publications/world_malaria_report_2013/report/en/. Accessed November 10, 2014

WHO. Chronic respiratory diseases: chronic obstructive pulmonary disease (COPD). Geneva: World Health Organization; 2014. Available at: http://www.who.int/respiratory/copd/en. Accessed November 10, 2014

WHO. Drowning. Fact sheet No. 347. Geneva: World Health Organization; 2014. Available at: http://www.who.int/mediacentre/factsheets/fs347/en/. Accessed November 10, 2014

WHO. Global Health Observatory Data Repository: welcome to global health workforce statistics. Available at http://apps.who.int/gho/data/node.main.HWF?lang=en. Accessed November 10, 2014

WHO. Global Status Report on Alcohol and Health 2014. Geneva: Wolrd Health Organization; 2014. Available at: http://www.who.int/substance_abuse/publications/global_alcohol_report/en/. Accessed November 10, 2014

WHO. Health statistics and information systems: global health estimates 2014 summary tables: deaths by cause, age and sex, by WHO region, 2000–2012. Geneva: World Health Organization; 2014. Available at: http://www.who.int/healthinfo/global_burden_disease/en/. Accessed November 10, 2014

WHO. Tobacco. Fact sheet No. 339. Geneva: World Health Organization; 2014. Available at: http://www.who.int/mediacentre/factsheets/fs339/en/. Accessed November 10, 2014

WHO. World Health Statistics 2014. Geneva: World Health Organization; 2014. Available at: http://apps.who.int/iris/bitstream/10665/112738/1/9789240692671_eng.pdf?ua=1.   Accessed November 30, 2014

World Directory of Medical Schools. 7th ed. Geneva: Harvard Business School Publishing; 2005

Wright G. Antibiotics: An irresistible newcomer. Nature. 2015;517:442–444

zur Hausen H. Zukunft der Krebsforschung. Frankfurt/Main: Campus; 1996

Abbreviations

ACE	angiotensin-converting enzyme
ACGME	Accreditation Council for Graduate Medical Education
AHRQ	Agency for Healthcare Research and Quality
AIDS	acquired immunodeficiency syndrome
ATP	adenosine triphosphate
BAL	British anti-Lewisite
BfArM	Bundesinstitut für Arzneimittel und Medizinprodukte (Germany)
BLS	basic life support
CCP	cyclic citrullinated peptide
COPD	chronic obstructive pulmonary disease
CT	computed tomography
DNA	deoxyribonucleic acid
DSM	*Diagnostic and Statistical Manual of Mental Disorders*
ECG	electrocardiogram/electrocardiographic
EDTA	ethylenediaminetetraacetic acid
EEG	electroencephalogram/electroencephalographic
e-learning	electronic learning
ERCP	endoscopic retrograde cholangiopancreatography
FACS	fluorescence-activated cell sorting
FDA	Food and Drug Administration (USA)
GABA	γ-aminobutyric acid
HIV	human immunodeficiency virus
HLA	human leukocyte antigen
HPV	human papillomavirus

ICD	*International Statistical Classification of Diseases and Related Health Problems*
LSD	lysergic acid diethylamide
MAO-B	monoamine oxidase B
MAOI	monoamine oxidase inhibitor
MRI	magnetic resonance imaging
NICE	National Institute for Health and Care Excellence (UK)
NRI	noradrenaline reuptake inhibitor
OECD	Organisation for Economic Co-operation and Development
PCR	polymerase chain reaction
PET-CT	positron emission tomography–computed tomography
SIRT	selective internal radiation therapy
SNRI	serotonin and noradrenaline reuptake inhibitor
SPECT	single photon emission–computed tomography
SSRI	selective serotonin reuptake inhibitor
TACE	transarterial chemoembolization
TNM	tumor–node–metastasis
UNAIDS	Joint United Nations Programme on HIV/AIDS
VATS	video-assisted thoracoscopic surgery
WHO	World Health Organization
WISC	Wechsler Intelligence Scale for Children

Short Biographies

Whatever may befall you,
it was preordained for you from everlasting.

Marcus Aurelius

Ackerknecht, Erwin Heinz, German–American ethnologist and medical historian, born in 1906 in Szczecin, Poland, and died in 1988 in Zurich, Switzerland. He is the author of *A Short History of Medicine* and other various standard references; he also wrote the biography of Rudolf Virchow. He was the director of the Institute of the History of Medicine at the University of Zurich and established its international reputation. He considered ethnologic and sociocultural aspects in his descriptions of diseases and his portrayal of medical history.

Addison, Thomas, British physician and university lecturer, born in 1793 in Longbenton, England, and died in 1860 in Brighton, England. He predominantly devoted himself to skin diseases, published descriptions of numerous diseases, and researched poisons. In 1855, he was the first to describe adrenocortical insufficiency, which was then named after him (Addison's disease).

Adler, Alfred, Austrian physician and psychotherapist, born in 1870 in Rudolfsheim near Vienna, Austria, and died in 1937 in Aberdeen, Scotland. He studied with Sigmund Freud; however, after their relationship broke down in 1911, he began his own research on "organ inferiority" and feelings of inferiority. This research culminated in his best-known work, *The Practice and Theory of Individual Psychology* (1924 in English). This "individual psychology" approach made him one of the most renowned Western psychologists. The theory of individual psychology still attracts considerable attention in modern times, particularly in the United States.

Barnard, Christiaan Neethling, South African heart surgeon and university lecturer, born in 1922 in Beaufort West, South Africa, and died in 2001 in Paphos, Cyprus. On December 3, 1967, he performed the world's first heart transplantation at the Groote Schuur Hospital in Cape Town, South Africa. The heart donor was Denise Ann Darvall; the heart recipient was Louis Washkansky, who lived for 18 days with the implanted heart. Barnard was an international headliner. In Austria, he founded a charity for underprivileged children that was named after him.

Bernard, Claude, French physiologist and university professor, born in 1813 in Saint-Julien, France, and died in 1878 in Paris, France. He discovered the functions of the pancreas in digestion and the function of the liver in glucose metabolism. He is considered to be one of the founders of experimental medicine. He was also the first person to describe the significance of the internal environment for preserving life.

Bleuler, Paul Eugen, Swiss psychiatrist, born in 1857 and died in 1939 in Zollikon, Switzerland. He denied the strict division between mental health and mental disease. He was one of the first clinical psychiatrists who supported psychoanalysis. He defined the terms *schizophrenia* and *autism*. He is the author of the 1916 publication, *Textbook of Psychiatry*, which became a standard reference for the field.

Cushing, Harvey Williams, American surgeon and university professor, born in 1869 in Cleveland, Ohio, and died in 1939 in New Haven, Connecticut. He is considered the most important neurosurgeon of the twentieth century and the founder of brain surgery. He was a pioneer in blood pressure readings and the diagnostic application of radiography. He also introduced anesthesia case logs and, in 1923, he established the first intensive care unit in medical history in Boston, Massachusetts.

Descartes, René, French philosopher, mathematician, and natural scientist, born in 1596 in La Haye en Touraine, France, and died in 1650 in Stockholm, Sweden. His rationalistic thinking founded the early modern rationalism movement and analytical geometry. Newton's laws of motion negated his scientific work, but his philosophy is effective to this day. His dictum "Cogito ergo sum," which roughly translates into "I think, therefore I am," sums up the core of Descartesian philosophy.

Ehrlich, Paul, German physician, serologist, pharmaceutical researcher, and university professor, born in 1854 in Strehlen near Wrocław, Poland, died in 1915 in Bad Homburg vor der Höhe, Germany. He examined the biochemical basics of immunity, discerned different types of blood cells, and, together with Emil von Behring, developed the antiserum used against diphtheria. In 1910, he introduced arsphenamine (Salvarsan), an arsenic-based drug and the first effective treatment for syphilis. It was also the first "blockbuster" drug in the world. He is considered to be the father of modern chemotherapy. In 1908, he shared the Nobel Prize in Physiology or Medicine with Ilja Iljitsch Metschnikow for his research in the field of immunity.

Fleming, Alexander, Scottish bacteriologist and university professor, born in 1881 in Lochfield, Scotland, and died in 1955 in London, England. He discovered lysozyme and the antiseptic effects of the mold fungus *Penicillium*. In 1945, he shared the Nobel Prize in Physiology or Medicine with Howard Walter Florey and Ernst Boris Chain for the development of the antibiotic penicillin.

Freud, Sigmund, Austrian psychoanalyst, neurologist, depth psychologist, born in 1856 in Příbor, Czech Republic, and died in 1939 in London, England. After experimenting with cocaine, hypnosis, and suggestion, he developed in conjunction with Josef Breuer the basics of "talk therapy." He was the founder of psychoanalysis, which brings subconscious and suppressed contents to consciousness via free associations and dream interpretation. By bringing causative issues to consciousness, he claimed to treat psychological disorders. Freud's briefest description of psychoanalytic techniques was: "Remember, repeat, and work through it."

Galen of Pergamon, Greco-Roman physician and anatomist, born between in 129 and 131 AD in Pergamon, Greece, died around in 199 or 216 AD in Rome. He became one of the most influential physicians during the Roman Empire by combining Hippocrates' humorism with anatomic insights he gained through animal dissection. He consolidated the entire ancient medicine in his 400 papers, which served as the foundation for medical teachings up until the sixteenth century.

Gebhardt, Ulrike, German science journalist and biologist, born in 1969 in Bremen, Germany. She regularly publishes articles on various bioscientific and medical topics in newspapers and professional magazines.

Geisler, Linus S., German physician, university professor and publicist, born in 1934 in Vyškovce, Slovakia. His specialties include internal medicine, contemporary bioethical issues, and physician–patient communication.

Gram, Hans Christian Joachim, Danish bacteriologist and university professor, born in 1853 and died in 1938 in Copenhagen, Denmark. Between 1883 and 1885 he developed the most important medical dyeing method, which was named after him—the Gram stain. It is still used in modern times. The method allows for the differentiation between gram-positive and gram-negative bacteria based on the structure of the cell wall.

Graves, Robert James, Irish physician, born in 1796 and died in 1853 in Dublin, Ireland. He supported learning at the bedside to ensure the physician-to-be would not end up as "a practitioner who has never practiced." He emphasized the importance of research and was the first to take a person's pulse with the aid of a watch. In 1835, he described a combination of symptoms of an autoimmune disease affecting the thyroid, a condition that now shares his name (Graves' disease).

Harvey, William, English physician, embryologist, and anatomist, born in 1578 in Kent, England, and died in 1657 in London, England. In 1628, he published *Exercitatio Anatomica de Motu Cordis et Sanguinis in Animalibus* (Anatomical Studies on the Motions of the Heart and the Blood in Living Beings), in which he was the first person to describe a complete theory of blood circulation. He differentiated between hypotheses and facts, and introduced scientific methods to the fields of biology and medicine. He is considered to be a pioneer of modern physiology.

Hippocrates of Kos, considered one of the most famous physicians of antiquity, born around 460 BC on the Greek island of Kos and died around 370 BC in Larissa, Thessaly. He is also considered the father of medical science and the first modern physician due to his systematical observations. In his mind, diseases were the expression of defective mixtures of humors. He emphasized anamnesis and did not treat the disease but the person as a whole. He required physical and mental hygiene, integrity, caution, empathy, and analytic thinking from every physician. The Hippocratic Oath is the first known ethical guideline for the medical profession and serves to this day as the foundation for medical professional ethics.

Holmes, Thomas H., American psychiatrist and university professor, born in 1918 in Wayne, North Carolina, and died in 1988 in King, Washington. In 1967, he and Richard H. Rahe developed the Social Readjustment Rating Scale, also known as the Holmes and Rahe stress scale. This scale illustrates the extent of life-event stress.

Jaspers, Karl Theodor, German–Swiss philosopher, physician, and psychiatrist, born in 1883 in Oldenburg, Germany, and died in 1969 in Basel, Switzerland. Aside from Martin Heidegger, he is considered the most significant proponent of German existentialism. He made essential contributions to the development of psychiatry. In 1958, he was awarded the Peace Prize of the German Book Trade for his critical sociopolitical commitment.

Jellinek, Elvin Morton, American physiologist and university professor, born in 1890 in New York, and died in 1963 in Palo Alto, California. He was the first person to recognize the disease pattern of alcoholism and developed a five-stage classification for people with alcohol problems. He designed a questionnaire to evaluate the presence of alcoholism and its stages.

Jenner, Edward Anthony, English physician, born in 1749 and died in 1823 in Berkeley, England. In 1796 he developed the first reliable procedure of immunization with poxvirus called a "vaccination." Up until then, immunization was only practiced as a risky preventive measure. It was Jenner who discovered that a cuckoo pushes its "step-siblings" out of the nest. The lunar crater Jenner was named after him.

Kant, Immanuel, German philosopher of the Enlightenment, and possibly the most influential thinker of occidental philosophy, born in 1724 and died in 1804 in Königsberg, East Prussia. In 1781, he published *Critique of Pure Reason*, in which he overcame the rationalism and empiricism of his time. His critical and transcendental philosophy became the foundation of modern philosophy. Common knowledge was his categorical imperative. He defined the Enlightenment movement as "man's emergence from his self-imposed nonage… Dare to know!"

Koch, Heinrich Hermann Robert, German physician and microbiologist, born in 1843 in Clausthal-Zellerfeld, Germany, and died in 1910 in Baden-Baden, Germany. Next to Louis Pasteur, he is considered one of the founders of bacteriology and microbiology. He was the first to cultivate the splenic fever pathogen outside of a host, discovered the tuberculosis pathogen, and developed the putative cure tuberculin. He instituted tropical medicine and realized the importance of hygiene for health. In 1905, he was awarded the Nobel Prize in Physiology or Medicine.

Kuebler-Ross, Elisabeth, Swiss–American psychiatrist and university professor, born in 1926 in Zurich, Switzerland, and died in 2004 in Scottsdale, Arizona. She devoted her work to the studies of death and grieving. In 1969, her *On Death and Dying* was published and laid the foundation for thanatology. Alongside Cicely Saunders, she is considered to be one of the initiators of the hospice movement and self-help groups for grieving persons.

Major, Johann Daniel, German physician and polymath, born in 1634 in Wrocław, Poland, and died in 1693 in Stockholm, Sweden. He founded museology and performed the first public dissections of executed criminals in Northern Germany. Next to Christopher Wren, he is considered to be the inventor of intravenous injections; however, he was convinced of the usefulness of injections in drug therapy, whereas Wren was not.

McMoran Wilson, Charles, English physician, born in 1882 in Skipton, England, and died in 1977 in Newton Valence, England. As the dean of London's St. Mary's Hospital Medical School and the president of the Royal College of Physicians, he became the personal physician to Winston Churchill and wrote the book *Winston Churchill – The Struggle for Survival 1940–1965* in 1966. Both Churchill and the book made him a public figure. He also played a decisive role in the Britain's National Health Service Constitution.

Meerwein, Fritz, Swiss psychiatrist, psychoanalyst, and president of the Swiss Society for Psychoanalysis, born in 1922 in Basel, Switzerland, and died in 1989 in Heidelberg, Germany. He devoted himself to psychosomatics and psychological issues in oncologic diseases and is considered to be the pioneer of psycho-oncology.

Milgram, Stanley, American psychologist and university lecturer, born in 1933 and died in 1984 in New York. He became known through his experiments on authority and obedience. These experiments showed the average person's willingness to follow authoritarian orders against their conscience. He also developed the small-world theory—colloquially known as "six degrees of separation"—claiming that any two people can be connected with a maximum of six steps (acquainted people) in between.

Mittler, Barbara, German sinologist, born in 1968 in Hagen, Germany. She is the head of the Institute for Sinology in Heidelberg, Germany. Her research is focused on public spheres, examining the cultural motion to and from China and their manifestations in different media.

Paracelsus (Philippus Aureolus Theoprastus Bombastus von Hohenheim), Swiss–German physician, alchemist, astrologist, mystic, and philosopher, born in 1493 or 1494 in Egg, Switzerland, and died in 1541 in Salzburg, Austria. He opposed the scholastic attitude in science and the prevailing teachings, such as Galen's humoral pathology. He confronted the submissiveness to authorities and written texts with observations taken from nature and findings from scientific experiments. Despite his legendary successes in healing, which became the foundation for modern pharmaceutical therapy, his approach was met by his contemporaries with animosity. His significance in the history of medicine was misjudged for many years.

Pasteur, Louis, French chemist, bacteriologist, and university professor, born in 1822 in Dole, France, and died in 1895 in Villeneuve l'Étang near Paris, France. He is considered to be a cofounder of microbiology due to his research on fermentation. He developed vaccines for fowl cholera, splenic fever, swine erysipelas, and rabies, as well as a method to kill microorganisms using heat, thus laying the groundwork for the process of pasteurization. In 1887, he founded an institute in Paris that still carries his name in modern times and is dedicated to bacterial research and vaccine development.

Penzoldt, Franz, German internist, pharmacologist, and university professor, born in 1849 in Crispendorf, Germany, and died in 1927 in Munich, Germany. He studied pediatrics and was the director of the Medical Institute in Erlangen, Germany, from 1903 until 1920. His *Textbook of Clinical Pharmaceutical Treatment for Students and Physicians* became a standard reference.

Rahe, Richard H., American psychiatrist and university professor, born in 1936 in Seattle, Washington. In 1967, in conjunction with Thomas H. Holmes, he developed the Social Readjustment Rating Scale, also known as the Holmes and Rahe stress scale, which illustrates the extent of life-event stress.

Ringel, Erwin, Austrian psychiatrist, neurologist, university professor, suicide researcher, and pioneer of psychosomatic medicine, born in 1921 in Timişoara, Romania, and died in 1994 in Bad Kleinkirchheim, Austria. In 1948, he established the first suicide prevention center in Vienna, Austria, which still stands today. From 1953 until 1964, he was the head of the women's section of the Psychiatric University Hospital in Vienna where he founded the first psychosomatic ward in Austria.

Roentgen, Wilhelm Conrad, German physicist, university professor, and principal of the University of Würzburg, born in 1845 in Lennep, Germany, and died in 1923 in Munich, Germany. In 1895 he discovered X-rays, which were then named after him. Roentgen rays revolutionized medical diagnostics. His discovery also influenced our knowledge about the atomic envelope, the crystalline grid structure, and the discovery of radioactivity. In 1901, he was awarded the first Nobel Prize in Physics. The 111th chemical element (roentgenium) and an asteroid are named after him.

Sauerbruch, Ernst Ferdinand, German surgeon, university professor, and hospital director, born in 1875 in Barmen, Germany, and died in 1951 in Berlin, Germany. His skills earned him the reputation as the most significant German surgeon of the twentieth century. He developed the hypobaric chamber, which allows surgery to take place at the open thorax. He also designed novel hand, arm, and leg prostheses. He improved procedures in cardiac, gastrointestinal, and esophageal surgeries that are still employed today.

Schadewaldt, Hans, German physician and medical historian, born in 1923 in Cottbus, Germany, and died in 2009 in Düsseldorf, Germany. He became well known for his research on the history of allergies. His specialties included marine and tropical medicine, hospital administration, and epidemics. Some of his publications became standard references in the medical field.

Schaefer, Hans, German physician and physiologist, born in 1906 in Düsseldorf, Germany, and died in 2000 in Heidelberg, Germany. He was cofounder of the Max Planck Society and director of the Physiological Institute of the University of Heidelberg and Institute for Labor and Community Medicine. He also served as a member for numerous associations as well as the council of the federal board of health (Bundesgesundheitsrat). He authored numerous publications that addressed economic and health care policies.

Schettler, Friedrich Gotthard, German internist, university professor, and clinic director, born in 1917 in Falkenstein, Germany, and died in 1996 in Heidelberg, Germany. His research focused on fat metabolism. Early on, he emphasized the significance of cholesterol with regard to changes of the vascular walls and is considered to be a pioneer in arteriosclerosis research. His textbooks on internal medicine have become standard references.

Semmelweis, Ignaz Philipp, Hungarian gynecologist and obstetrician, born in 1818 in Budapest, Hungary, and died in 1865 in Oberdöbling near Vienna, Austria. Known as the "savior of mothers," he discovered the infectious cause of childbed fever (puerperal fever) and tried to introduce proper protection and preventive measures such as handwashing; however, he failed to do so due to the resistance of his colleagues and his practice earned widespread acceptance only years after his death. The Semmelweis reflex, named after him, describes the spontaneous rejection of a novel idea without reflection that contradicts the prevailing opinion.

Sydenham, Thomas, English physician and psychiatrist, born in 1624 in Wynford Eagle near Dorchester, England, and died in 1689 in London, England. He is considered one of the founders of clinical medicine and epidemiology. He is sometimes called the "English Hippocrates" because of his thorough observation of symptoms and deduced therapeutic conclusions. His research focused on epilepsy and hysteria. In 1683, he was the first person to describe gout. Chorea minor is named after him (Sydenham's chorea).

van **Leeuwenhoek, Antonie**, born in 1632 and died in 1723 in Delft in the Netherlands. Van Leeuwenhoek, known as the father of microbiology, discovered "protozoa" – the single-celled organisms he called "animalcules". He also improved the microscope and laid the foundation for microbiology. He is often cited as the first microbiologist to study muscle fibers, bacteria, spermatozoa and blood flow in capillaries.

Vesalius, Andreas, Flemish physician, anatomist, and university professor, born in 1514 in Brussels, Belgium, and died in 1564 in Zakynthos, Greece. He was the personal physician to Emperor Charles V and Philipp II of Spain. He is known for performing public dissections. In 1543, his richly illustrated anatomical atlas *De Humani Corporis Fabrica* (The Fabric of the Human Body) was published, which was the beginning of modern anatomy and morphologic thinking in medicine. Vesalius prepared the skeleton of a notorious criminal he stole from the gallows for illustrative purposes. Called the "Basel Skeleton" it is now displayed at the Anatomical Museum in the University of Basel, Switzerland.

Virchow, Rudolf Ludwig Karl, German physician, archeologist, anthropologist, and liberal politician, born in 1821 in Świdwin, Poland, and died in 1902 in Berlin, Germany. He described the pathogenesis of thrombosis and in 1845 was the first to define leukemia. His theory of cellular pathology made him the founder of modern pathology. In his role as social reformer and hygienist, he devoted himself to primary medical care for the people, helped establish testing procedures for *Trichinella*, and helped to establish local hospitals.

von Auenbrugger, Joseph Leopold, Austrian physician, born in 1722 in Graz, Austria, and died in 1809 in Vienna, Austria. In 1761, he described percussion as an examination technique, which is used today. When he was a child, he learned from his father, a wine merchant, how to discern between liquid and gaseous contents of wine barrels through percussion. By tapping on the body's surface, the underlying tissue begins to vibrate, and the resulting qualities of the vibrations will indicate the condition of the tissue.

von Basedow, Carl Adolph, German physician and district medical officer, born in 1799 in Dessau, Germany, and died in 1854 in Merseburg, Germany. In 1840, he was the first person in the German-speaking world to describe hyperthyroidism; the condition was then named after him. He fought for hygiene and preventive health care, initiated examinations of drinking water, designed a disease registration form, and published about 60 scientific articles.

von Behring, Emil Adolf, German bacteriologist, serologist, and university professor, born in 1854 in Hansdorf, West Prussia, and died in 1917 in Marburg, Germany. Beginning in 1890, together with Paul Ehrlich, he developed an antiserum to be used against diphtheria, which, at that time, was one of the most frequent causes of death in children. Later, he did the same for tetanus, labeling him the father of serum therapy. In 1901, he was the first person to receive the Nobel Prize in Physiology or Medicine.

Wachsmuth, Werner, German surgeon, medical officer, and university professor, born in 1900 in Rostock, Germany, and died in 1990 in Würzburg, Germany. From 1940 to 1944, he was the head of the army surgical hospital in Brussels, Belgium, and traveled to the war zones with his mentor Ferdinand Sauerbruch. Between 1946 and 1969 he was the chair for surgery at the Julius Maximilians University in Würzburg.

Wesiack, Wolfgang, Austrian physician, professor, and psychoanalyst, born in 1924 in Graz, Austria, and died in 2013 in Göppingen, Germany. In collaboration with Thure von Uexküll, he developed the foundations of psychosomatic medicine. He was a professor of medical psychology and psychotherapy and devoted himself to the development of the physician–patient relationship.

Wren, Christopher, English astronomer and architect, born 1632 in East Knoyle, England, and died in 1723 in Hope under Dinmore, England. After the Fire of London in 1666, he was became the Surveyor General of the King's Works. Wren designed more than 60 churches and public buildings, which included Kensington Palace and St. Paul's Cathedral. In 1656, he performed the first intravenous injection on a canine.

zur Hausen, Harald, German physician, born in 1936 in Gelsenkirchen, Germany. He researched the evolution of cancer due to viral infections and discovered the association between human papillomavirus and cervical cancer. In 2008, he was awarded the Nobel Prize in Physiology or Medicine.

Figure Sources

Figs. 3.1; 3.3	Kahle W, Frotscher M. Color Atlas of Human Anatomy, Vol. 3: Nervous System and Sensory Organs. 7th ed. Stuttgart–New York: Thieme Publishers; 2015
Figs. 3.2; 3.6; 3.16; 3.24; 3.25	Fritsch H, Kuehnel W. Color Atlas of Human Anatomy, Vol. 2: Internal Organs. 6th ed. Stuttgart–New York: Thieme Publishers; 2015
Figs. 3.4; 3.5a,b; 3.7; 3.13a	Steffers G, Credner S. General Pathology and Internal Medicine for Physical Therapists. Stuttgart–New York: Thieme Publishers; 2012
Fig. 3.8	Garcia-Elias M, Mathoulin C. Articular Injury of the Wrist. Stuttgart–New York: Thieme Publishers; 2014
Fig. 3.9	Block B. Abdominal Ultrasound. 3rd ed. Stuttgart–New York: Thieme Publishers; 2016
Fig. 3.10	Lapp H, Krakau I. The Cardiac Catheter Book. Stuttgart–New York: Thieme Publishers; 2014
Figs. 3.11; 3.12; 3.21	Kirchner J. Chest Radiology: A Resident's Manual. Stuttgart–New York: Thieme Publishers; 2011
Figs. 3.13b; 3.14; 3.15a-c; 3.20	Siegenthaler W. Differential Diagnosis in Internal Medicine. From Symptom to Diagnosis. Stuttgart–New York: Thieme Publishers; 2007
Fig. 3.17	Sterry W, Paus R, Burgdorf W. Thieme Clinical Companions: Dermatology. Stuttgart–New York: Thieme Publishers; 2006
Fig. 3.18	Rohkamm R. Color Atlas of Neurology. 2nd ed. Stuttgart–New York: Thieme Publishers; 2015
Fig. 3.22	Krischak G. Traumatology for the Physical Therapist. Stuttgart–New York: Thieme Publishers; 2014
Fig. 3.23	Schnettler R. Septic Bone and Joint Surgery. Stuttgart–New York: Thieme Publishers; 2010
Fig. 3.26	Lang G. Opthalmology. Stuttgart–New York: Thieme Publishers; 2006
Fig. 3.27	Georgalas C, Fokkens W. Rhinology and Skull Base Surgery. From the Lab to the Operating Room: An Evidence-based Approach. Stuttgart–New York: Thieme Publishers; 2013

Index